FROM PULPIT...

...TO COUCH

RABBI
ABRAHAM J. TWERSKI, M.D.

MIRKOV PUBLICATIONS, INC.
PITTSBURGH, PENNSYLVANIA

MIRKOV PUBLICATIONS, INC.
P.O. Box 81971
Pittsburgh, Pennsylvania 15217
1-(800)-851-8303
WWW.MIRKOV.COM

Copyright © 2005 by Abraham J. Twerski

Library of Congress Control Number: 2005923736

10 9 8 7 6 5 4 3 2 1

All rights reserved. Printed in the United States of America. No part of this book may be reproduced or copied in any manner or in any medium whatsoever without written permission from Mirkov Publications, Inc. except in the case of brief quotations in reviews for inclusion in a magazine, newspaper or broadcast.

ISBN 0-9766337-0-1

Manufactured in the United States of America

TABLE OF CONTENTS

PREFACE
INTRODUCTION 12
THE IMPORTANCE OF LEARNING 15

LESSONS FROM RECOVERY

MY TEACHER, ISABEL 18
REFRESHINGLY SIMPLE 24
THE SPIRITUALITY DEFICIENCY SYNDROME 27
START ROWING, THE BOAT WILL APPEAR 30
WHEN YOU CAN'T MAKE AMENDS 32
THE TOXICITY OF RESENTMENTS 34

COPING

IT'S GOING TO TURN OUT O.K. 38
ACCEPTING A DIFFICULT REALITY 41
WELCOME DISCOMFORT 45
CAN THERE BE JOY IN HURTING? 47
A REFRESHER COURSE 49
THE PAIN OF LEARNING 51
NOTHING TO FEAR BUT FEAR 53
WHY CRY WHEN YOU CAN LAUGH? 55
GRATITUDE 57
GOD NEVER DESERTS 59
LET GO AND LET GOD 61
MANY WORRIES? BE HAPPY! 63

SOME ANNOYANCES ARE GOOD FOR YOU	64
WE KNOW WHOM WE CAN TRUST	65
USE AND DISCARD	67
EVEN A BAD FALL IS JUST A FALL	69
STAY WITHIN REALITY	71
FROM HORSES AND SALMON	72

THERAPEUTIC TECHNIQUES

HOW TO LISTEN	74
A SIMPLE FORMULA	76
TRANSFERENCE AND COUNTER-TRANSFERENCE	78
WHAT A PLUMBER TAUGHT ME	80
TO TELL THE TRUTH	82
THE THERAPIST'S CONVICTIONS	84
PSYCHOTHERAPY OF PSYCHOSIS	86
ABSURD PROBLEMS MAY BE DISMISSED	89

SELF AWARENESS AND SELF ESTEEM

SEEKING AN IDENTITY	92
TO BE ALWAYS TEACHABLE	94
TO BE FREE	96
FORGIVING OURSELVES	98

FROM LITERATURE

EVEN GREAT MINDS ARE NOT INFINITE	101
"DOCTOR" CHARLES SCHULZ	103
THE DISCOMFORT ZONE	106

FROM PEERS AND FRIENDS

DON'T TREAT HEALTH	109
SMILING IS GOOD FOR YOU	111
WHEN SELFISHNESS IS GOOD	112
A WISE GUIDELINE	113
AGING HAS ITS ADVANTAGES	114
DON'T JUMP TO CONCLUSIONS	116
A HELPFUL HINT	118
INSANE OR NORMAL?	119

…AND FROM PATIENTS

DEATH IS ALWAYS SUDDEN	122
LOVE AND LIKE ARE NOT SYNONYMOUS	124
TO BE ALWAYS CONSIDERATE	125
THE BEAUTY OF LIGHT	126
DIAMONDS	128
AFRAID OF PRAISE	131
BEWARE THE LABELING	132
ACCEPTING HELP	133
MARRIAGE COUNSELING	134
DEPRESSED ABOUT?	135
WHAT ELSE IS THERE?	136
THE NEED FOR AN IDENTITY	138

STORIES

BRIEF PSYCHOTHERAPY	**140**
ENTERING THE WORLD OF THE PSYCHOTIC	**144**
CLOSED - MINDEDNESS	**146**
NEVER SATISFIED	**149**
IT'S HOW YOU SEE IT	**152**
TO WIN AN ARGUMENT	**154**
THE WAY OF BUREAUCRACY	**155**
THE PURSUIT OF HAPPINESS	**156**

DEDICATED TO ALL MY TEACHERS

PREFACE

FROM PULPIT TO PULPIT (VIA COUCH)

There was never any doubt in my mind what I was going to be when I grew up. I was going to be a rabbi like my father.

My father was a Hasidic rabbi, with uncanny, innate psychological acumen and keen knowledge of the ways of the world that made him a much sought after counselor. In addition he was so successful as a mediator that judges would say, "Take this case to Twerski." My father received a citation from the Milwaukee judiciary.

My father's study was always humming, day and night, with people who sought his advice and guidance. I wanted to be just like him.

When I was ordained in 1951, I became his assistant. In the years following World War II, psychiatry and psychology had a meteoric rise. It was fashionable to be psychoanalyzed. It became obvious to me that in contrast to my father, people were not going to consult me for anything. It was not primarily because I was still wet behind the ears, but rather because the competence for counseling was felt to be with the professional psychotherapist rather than with the clergy. Pastoral psychology had not yet come into its own.

Nor did people seem to be interested in adult education. I would have loved to teach, but there were no students, except those coming for bar-mitzvah classes, and they all "graduated" at 13.

My function as a rabbi was to officiate at weddings, bar-mitzvahs, funerals, monument dedications and other rituals. I saw my life as being one of a performer of ceremonies rather than as teacher or counselor, and this was hardly to my liking. It was evident that if I wanted to function as the kind of rabbi my father was, I'd have to become a psychiatrist or psychologist. That led me to follow a medical career at Milwaukee's Marquette University.

After a year's internship in general medicine, I underwent three years of training in psychiatry at the University of Pittsburgh.

I was the fair-haired boy of the Director of the Department of Psychiatry, who promised me a staff position after completing two years service at a state mental hospital.

When I returned, the director said, "Abe, I promised you a staff position, and you can have it. But I want you to consider the directorship of St. Francis Hospital's psychiatric service. St. Francis has been the largest provider of community psychiatric services, and they have not been able to keep a director. The community owes St. Francis a debt, and I want you to consider the position. Try it for a year."

Simply to satisfy the chief, I met with Sister Adele, St. Francis Hospital's administrator. I gave her numerous reasons why I was not the person for the position, but Sister was adamant. Upon leaving, Sister escorted me all the way and said, "Dr. Twerski, I know you will come to us. The Holy Ghost sent you to us."

I wanted to be in the chief's good graces, so I took the job for a year after which I would go back to the university. That year extended itself to *twenty* years.

St. Francis had a large alcohol-detoxification service, because many hospitals rejected alcoholics as well as mentally ill patients as undesirables. As you will soon see, I had become interested in the 12-step program for alcoholism recovery. I realized that simply "drying-out" the alcoholic was not enough, and I prevailed upon Sister to develop a residential rehabilitation center. In 1972, Gateway Rehabilitation Center admitted its first patient. Today, it is a rehabilitation "system," providing services to 1800 people on an average day.

A frequently asked question is, "Did the training and experience as a rabbi affect your practice of psychiatry?" Of course it did. Every experience one has impacts on one's thinking and behavior. Certainly my religious training gave me insights into spirituality, although, as you shall see, it is possible to be spiritual even if one has no religious orientation.

The most profound effect of my earlier life in religion was greatly influenced by my father's staunch conviction of the inherent good in man (albeit there are some exceptions). When someone referred to a person as being bad, my father would say,

"He is not really bad, he is foolish. He does not understand that what he is doing is self-destructive. How can I bear a grudge against someone when I pity him for being a fool?" So, much of my success in treating alcoholics and drug addicts is due to my belief that they are inherently good people.

The struggle of the alcoholic and drug-addict to break free of their addiction is a model for everyone who wishes to improve one's spiritual life. So, although no longer officiating as a rabbi, I feel myself very much to be a rabbi, with my patients as my congregants. "Rabbi" means "teacher," and I have been blessed to be able to teach people about their self-worth. To do what he excelled at, my father became a rabbi, and I emulated him by becoming a psychiatrist.

INTRODUCTION

"Who is a wise person? One who learns from everyone"
(Talmud)

My formal education began at age five, when I was taught my first words of the Torah. My formal religious education continued until I was ordained at age twenty-one. During my ten years as a pulpit rabbi, I continued my studies on my own.

A new path in learning came with medical school, followed by three years of psychiatric training. The chief of our department wisely added major literary works to the curriculum. In addition to psychiatric texts, we had a weekly literature seminar featuring the works of Dostoevsky, Tolstoy, Thomas Mann, Melville and other great authors. Freud once said that Dostoevsky knew more about the workings of the unconscious mind than all of the psychoanalytic congress put together.

In this wide world, we can learn from everyone and everything. Rabbi Israel of Salant was once walking with several disciples when he saw a procession of three horse-drawn wagons loaded with hay. The middle horse was eating the hay from the wagon in front of him, and the third horse was eating from the middle wagon.

"What does that teach you?" Rabbi Israel asked his students. When there was no reply, he said, "The horse pulling the first wagon has nothing to eat, but he does benefit because his load becomes lighter as the horse behind him eats. The load of the third horse does not become any lighter, but he can eat from the middle wagon. The middle horse has the greatest benefit, because he can eat from the wagon in front of him and his load becomes lighter as the horse behind him eats from his wagon.

"This teaches you that the greatest benefit is accrued by one who takes a middle-of-the-road approach and avoids either extreme."

If we keep an open mind, we can learn from things we see in the street, even from horses. I was fortunate in being exposed to people and things from whom I could learn, and this substantially supplemented what I received from formal training, both as a psychiatric physician and as a rabbi.

Psychologists and psychiatrists learn a great deal in their training. However, I recall the words of Paracelsus, a sixteenth century physician in Switzerland, who assembled his medical students around a huge bonfire and threw all the medical books into the fire. "If you want to learn medicine," he said, "go study your patients."

Fortunately, that is no longer true. Our modern textbooks contain a great deal of valuable information. Nevertheless, it is still true that we learn most from our patients. There is just no substitute for experience. Psychiatrists and psychologists are always educable, always alert to what they may learn from their patients, unless of course, they close their minds to anything new.

In psychiatry, as in other fields of medicine, we must learn new things as our science progresses. We must also be able to *unlearn* some things.

In addition to learning from my patients and from the masters of classic literature, I also found profound psychological insights in the cartoons of Charles Schulz, creator of Snoopy and Charlie Brown. This resulted in the publication of several books on Schulz's insights. In fact, I was able to develop a system of "cartoon therapy." I found that some patients who were resistive to my interpretations could accept them when they saw themselves in the cartoon characters.

I was also privileged to hear many stories from my patients from which I could derive valuable psychotherapeutic tools. There is much wisdom in folk tales and folklore.

Forty years of attending meetings of Alcoholics Anonymous provided a common sense approach to many of the problems of life. My teachers were people who, having discarded the futile attempt to escape from life's problems by drinking or using drugs, had developed effective skills for coping with difficulties.

Long-term, quality recovery from alcoholism is impossible without development of spirituality. Working with people in recovery actually intensified my pursuit of spirituality that I had begun as a rabbi.

I take this opportunity to share with you some of the wisdom that was made available to me.

THE IMPORTANCE OF LEARNING

Obviously, learning is important. But in addition to the expedience of greater knowledge and wisdom, there is another reason.

Some people have a misconception about spirituality. They think that a highly spiritual person is a self-flagellating ascetic, someone who has isolated himself from people and lives a contemplative life in the forest, praying all day.

The rabbi of Rhizin confronted a young man who had come to learn from him. "What progress have you made in your spirituality?" he asked.

The young man answered, "Rabbi, I have avoided eating anything but the simplest food. I make penance for my sins by putting nails in my shoes and having someone give me forty lashes once a week. I have also taken a vow to keep silent half a day."

The rabbi took the young man by the hand and led him to the barn. "See that horse?" he said. "He eats only the simplest food, has nails in his shoes, receives many more than forty lashes a week, and is silent *all* day. But he's still a horse."

What *is* spirituality?

The human being is a composite creature, comprised of a body + something else. Our body is essentially an animal body, and what makes us distinct and unique as human beings is that "something else," which consists of those things that animals do not have.

Some of the more obvious uniquely human features are: (1) greater intelligence, (2) the ability to learn from the history of past generations, (3) the ability to reflect on the purpose and goals of life, (4) the ability to volitionally improve oneself, (5) the ability to think about future consequences of one's actions, (6) the ability to defy bodily drives and make moral and ethical choices and (7) the ability to empathize with others and be considerate, etc. I'm sure you can come up with many more traits that people have that are not present in animals in the wild.

I group all these together and say that *the sum total of all the traits that are unique to humans is what we may refer to as the "spirit"*. These are all uniquely human *abilities*. If a person implements these traits and puts these abilities into action, one is implementing one's spirit, and this makes one *spiritual*.

The first of these traits is "greater intelligence." We increase our intelligence only by learning. Since increasing our intelligence is so significant a human trait, it is important that we be able to learn from everyone.

Spirituality does not require detachment from the world. Spirituality is simply being the finest human being one can be. We can always become better people, better for ourselves and better for others, but only by learning.

I found that in their addiction, alcoholics lost much spirituality. They did not learn from the past, did not search for meaning in life, did not seek to improve their humanity, did not delay gratification, did not think of the consequences of their behavior, and they were not free. Alcohol is a cruel taskmaster when it has someone in its clutches. In recovery, alcoholics had to improve upon their spirituality.

You may have noticed that I have not included religion as part of spirituality. If a person strives to be the best person he can be, he may be spiritual even if he is not religion-oriented. Religion comes in when one begins to think about an ultimate purpose in life, and may find it in religion.

What is there one can learn from recovering alcoholics? Let's see.

LESSONS FROM RECOVERY

Out of suffering come the strongest souls: God's wounded often make His best soldiers.

Geraldine O. Delaney

MY TEACHER, ISABEL

I learned many things at meetings of Alcoholics Anonymous. Inasmuch as I never drank, why did I attend meetings of AA? Here's how it happened.

I was in my second year of psychiatric training when I received a call from the psych emergency room. A woman said she had to see a psychiatrist promptly and could not wait for an appointment.

Isabel was sixty-one. She was one of three daughters of an Episcopalian priest. Isabel began drinking late in adolescence, and at twenty she was into very heavy drinking. She married and had a child. When the child was three, her husband said, "Make your choice. It's either the booze or the family." "I knew I could not stop drinking," Isabel said, "and I wasn't much of a wife or mother. It was only decent to give him the divorce he asked for."

At sixty-one, Isabel was still attractive, and she must have been stunning at twenty-eight. Free and unattached, she began serving as an escort to some of Pittsburgh's social elite. She had a beautiful apartment, the latest in fashions, and all the alcohol she wanted.

After five years, the alcohol began to cause behavioral changes that made Isabel undesirable company for her clientele. She then began serving a lower socio-economic clientele, and very rapidly deteriorated. She was soon living in flea-bag hotels and prostituting.

Every so often, Isabel was found passed-out from drinking and taken to a hospital for detoxification. She attended the AA meetings in the hospital, and upon discharge promptly resumed drinking. When I assumed the position as director of psychiatry at St. Francis Hospital, I looked up Isabel's record. Between 1938 and 1956, Isabel had been detoxed at this hospital 59 times! At another hospital that offered detox she had 22 admissions. I was unable to get any information from other hospitals where she had undergone detoxification.

Isabel's family was horrified by her behavior and disowned her. Her phone calls to her sisters were answered with a brusque, "Don't you dare call me again," and a hang-up.

In 1956, Isabel approached a lawyer who had helped her out of some alcohol-related jams. "David, I need a favor," she said.

"Good God!" the lawyer said. "Not again! What did you do this time?"

"I'm not in any trouble," Isabel said. "I want you to put me away in the state hospital for a year."

At that time Pennsylvania statutes had an Inebriate Act, under which a chronic alcoholic could be committed to a state hospital for "a year and one day." This law had been used by families who wanted to get a chronic alcoholic out of their hair. No alcoholic had ever asked to be put away for a year.

"You don't know what you're asking for," the lawyer said. "You're crazy."

"If I'm crazy, I really belong in the state hospital," Isabel said. Isabel continued to press her request, and the lawyer finally took her before the judge and had her committed to the state hospital.

After a year of sobriety, Isabel left the state hospital and promptly went to an AA meeting. Someone gave her a few nights of shelter, and she soon found a job as a housekeeper for a nationally renowned physician.

The doctor was retired and was a chronic alcoholic. Many times Isabel had to lift him off the floor and put him in bed. He sat on the boards of several foundations and was periodically called to testify at Senate hearings. Isabel would receive a call from the doctor's children, "Dad has to be in Washington in two weeks. Get him into shape." Isabel would detox the doctor, get him a haircut and shave, and put him on the plane to Washington. "Now don't you drink on the plane or in Washington," she said. "When you come back tomorrow, I'll be waiting for you with a bottle." The doctor obeyed like a well-trained puppy.

I had never heard anything like this before. My first career was as a rabbi, and seminary did not teach me anything about alcoholism. Medical school was no better. I learned much about some rare diseases but nothing about the most common disease a doctor encounters. In my psychiatric training I was learning much about mental illnesses, but alcohol and drugs were never mentioned.

I was so fascinated by Isabel's story that I neglected to ask her what was the acute emergency. As a fledgling psychiatrist, I knew that there had to be motivation for a person to seek help. What could possibly have motivated Isabel to take so drastic a measure, to put herself into a state mental hospital for a year by a court order? I had to discover her reason, so I told her to come back in a week for another session.

In the next session I heard some more interesting stories. Inasmuch as I did not have a clue about her motivation, I had her come back the following week. To make a long story short, I saw Isabel once a week for thirteen years. One night, at age seventy-four, she died peacefully in her sleep.

I was curious how she was managing to stay sober. It was obvious to me that medicine and psychiatry had no effective treatment for alcoholism. What was her secret?

"I go to meetings of Alcoholics Anonymous," she said. In 1961, none of the celebrities had revealed that they were recovering alcoholics. Few people outside of AA knew anything about it.

"What happens at these meetings?" I asked. ""Who provides the treatment?"

"We have speakers meetings and discussion meetings, and we share our experiences," Isabel said.

"Do you have psychiatrists or psychologists there?" I asked.

Isabel said, "There is one psychologist who shows up occasionally, but he's still drunk most of the time."

"Look, Isabel," I said. "Some kind of treatment must be going on at these meetings if they are keeping you sober. Can I come and see for myself?"

"Sure," Isabel said. That week she took me to my first AA meeting.

The first thing that struck me at the meeting was that there was no stratification. Everyone was equal. No one could become president of the organization, and furthermore, money could not buy any special privileges.

As a synagogue rabbi, part of my job was to raise funds to cover the annual budget. Money came from the congregants' donations. People of lesser means made smaller contributions, and wealthier people made substantial contributions. I liked everyone equally, but I had to handle the large donors with silk gloves. I could not risk offending them, lest they leave for another congregation. Wealthy congregants received special treatment.

It is said that "Before God, everyone is equal." God can afford to treat everyone equally. He doesn't have to make mortgage payments each month. I did.

Any organization that is dependent on contributions is in the same situation. People with money or political clout are given preferential treatment. What impressed me about AA was that once people entered the room, everyone was equal. The rich received no special attention. Sometimes a poor person was in the position to help a wealthy person. Nor did academic status count. A fifth grade drop-out and a PhD were treated equally. I had never encountered anything like this!

Here is an example of AA's independence. I received a call from a man who said that he wanted to make a contribution of $10,000 to AA in memory of his late sister, who had enjoyed fourteen years of sobriety with the help of AA. He asked me where to send the check.

I called several people in AA, and when no one could help me, I called the AA central office. "Don't send the check here," they said. "We can't do anything with it."

"Then how can this man make a contribution?" I asked.

"He can cash the check at the bank and go to a meeting. When they pass the basket, he can put the money in."

"You want him to put $10,000 in cash in the basket?" I asked.

"Yes," was the answer. "But if he's not in the program, they might return it to him."

Never before and never since have I come across an organization that refuses donations.

My fascination with AA brought me back to more meetings. As I became familiar with the twelve steps for recovery, I concluded that they are much more than a method to stop drinking. They are a formula for mature, responsible living. There was nothing unique about alcoholics that made the twelve steps specific for them. I found that virtually every character defect that can be found in alcoholics can also be found in non-alcoholics, albeit they may be less pronounced. The twelve steps were a way for proper living, and I could apply them to myself.

So began my involvement with AA. I have attended meetings in many cities in the United States and in many countries I have visited. I can find friends in a community where I do not know a single person.

I would like to share with you some of what I have learned from AA. In case you happen to be a recovering person who thinks that all AA can do is keep you from drinking, you are missing out on a great deal of valuable knowledge.

What about the secret of Isabel's motivation to put herself into a state hospital? I never did solve that mystery in the thirteen years of therapy. I was left to my own devices to guess at it, and here is what I think.

Do you know how a volcano is formed? Deep down at the core of the earth, there is melted rock that is under extreme pressure. Over many centuries, this lava slowly makes its way through fissures in the earth's crust to the surface. Once it breaks through the surface, the lava erupts.

I believe that at the core of every human being there is a nucleus of self-respect and dignity. For a variety of reasons, this nucleus may be concealed and suppressed. Like the lava, it seeks to break through the surface and be recognized. Once it breaks through into a person's awareness, one may feel, "I am too good to be acting this way. This behavior is beneath my dignity." I think this is the "spiritual awakening" to which the twelfth step refers.

I think that this is what happened to Isabel. For years she had been blind to her self-worth and saw nothing wrong with her alcoholic behavior. Then one day, the nucleus of self-respect that had been buried deep within her broke through the surface, and she realized that she had no right to demean herself.

Why the state hospital? Let me share a personal experience.

I do most of my writing early in the morning when my mind is rested. One time the publisher told me that they were moving up the publishing date and that I had to complete the book sooner. That meant that I had to get up an hour earlier.

I set my alarm clock for 4:30. When it rang, I did what most people would do: I turned it off for just five minutes more of sleep. Of course, I woke up two hours later.

Several months later, I had to deliver a lecture in Washington, D.C. at 10 AM, which required my taking a 7 AM flight. To make this flight I had to be up at 5 AM. I set the alarm clock for 5 AM, but remembering my tendency to turn it off for "just five minutes" more of sleep, I realized that I might miss my flight. I took the alarm clock off the night stand and set it in the far corner of the room so that I could not turn it off from the bed. The next morning I awoke at 5 AM and walked across the room to turn off the alarm. I was then able to stay awake and make the flight.

On both occasions I had an awakening. The first awakening did not last long, because I went back to sleep. The second time I did something to avoid going right back to sleep. I made the awakening last.

Some people may have a spiritual awakening, but it does not last. Isabel knew that unless she took some measure to make her awakening last, she was likely to revert to drinking. The only way she knew to keep her awakening alive was to put herself out of reach of alcohol for an extended period of time. In those days there were few rehabilitation centers. The state hospital was her only option.

I am indebted to Isabel for bringing me to the twelve step programs. What was the crisis that brought her to the emergency room that day? There was no crisis. Why then did she seek an emergency appointment just on the day I was on emergency duty? Perhaps she was sent there to introduce me to AA. But who could have sent her? Your guess is as good as mine.

Let me share with you some of the wisdom I have derived from Alcoholics Anonymous.

REFRESHINGLY SIMPLE

"God made man straight, but they (people) sought many calculations." (Ecclesiastes 7:29)

It is well known that some people derive much benefit from a psychological interview because as they relate the problem, they begin to see things to which they had been oblivious. Often, the psychotherapist may help them over their blind spots, and they may then find the solution to their problem. Sometimes, the solutions to our problems would be evident if we hadn't "sought many calculations" and complicated them.

One particularly refreshing observation was made by a gentleman who was sober for more than twenty years. He picked me up at the airport, and as we were en route to a lecture, he related the following:

"I'm having a lot of trouble with a newcomer," he said. "He can't seem to put any sober time together. This guy says to me, 'You mean that you haven't had a single drink for over twenty years'?

" 'Yep,' I said.

" 'What's the trick?' he asked. 'I can't get by without a drink for even a week.'

" I said, 'There's no trick. Every morning, when I wake up, I ask God to give me another day of sobriety. At night, before I go to sleep, I thank God for having given me another day of sobriety.'

"So this guy says, 'Well, how do you know it was God who gave you a day of sobriety?'

"I looked at him and said, 'You dumb s.o.b. I didn't ask anyone else!' "

What could be simpler?

Sometimes our thinking may be so befuddled that we don't even consider the obvious. Alcohol is not the only thing that may cloud our thought processes. Any of many emotions may render us oblivious to the obvious.

One man related that after he had been sober for several years, he felt that it was safe for him to attend a New Year party. "I wanted to see how ridiculous reasonable people acted when they got drunk. It would remind me of how stupid I must have appeared when I drank, and it would give me another reason why not to drink.

"The only real reason that this humiliating behavior doesn't discourage people from drinking is because they don't remember a thing," he said.

He continued, "When everyone was good and tanked up, I walked over and raised the thermostat. Pretty soon it became uncomfortably hot, and people began removing their jackets. I then raised the thermostat a few more degrees, and the men removed their neckties and opened their collars. The women looked for magazines with which to fan themselves. It was a riot! No one even thought to look at the thermostat."

Wouldn't you think that when the room feels hot, the first thing one would do is look at the setting on the thermostat?

In my early days as a psychiatrist, I would always take a careful history, searching for the emotional traumas that were the cause of the patient's symptoms. This often is indeed necessary, but when the problem is more one of a maladjustment to a life situation, I listen carefully for what the patient may be overlooking, and what is preventing him from seeing the reason for his difficulty.

Sometimes, a person resists recognizing the true source of his problem in the present, because to do so would necessitate making changes in his life style. We are creatures of habit, and we generally do not like to make changes. A person may, therefore, attribute his problem to events of the past, and resign himself to his condition because the past cannot be changed. In such cases, I sometimes utilize this cartoon.

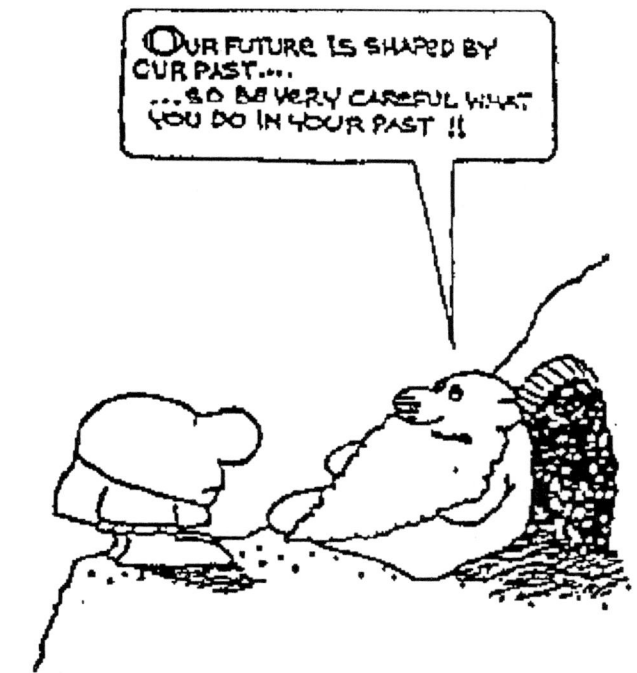

> OUR FUTURE IS SHAPED BY OUR PAST....
> ...SO BE VERY CAREFUL WHAT YOU DO IN YOUR PAST!!

ZIGGY © ZIGGY AND FRIENDS, INC. REPRINTED WITH PERMISSION OF UNIVERSAL PRESS SYNDICATE. ALL RIGHTS RESERVED

Ziggy's oracle is very wise. Inasmuch as we cannot change the past, it is sometimes better that we leave it alone and address the facts of the present.

I may also show a patient a comic strip where Linus tells Charlie Brown that we should not be so concerned about the future and just take care of today. Charlie Brown responds, "No, that would be giving up. I'm trying to make yesterday better." Patients can see the impossibility of this in the comic strip, and they may then be able to apply it to themselves.

Paying attention to what we are doing in the present is helpful in everyday life as well as in therapy. Sometimes we may not realize what may be the real cause of our discontent. We may have a deficiency of which we may not be aware, as the next piece suggests.

THE SPIRITUALITY DEFICIENCY SYNDROME

I got an important insight from listening to a veteran in alcoholism recovery, named Clancy.

After several decades of recovery in the program, Clancy gave his views on alcoholism. He said, "If your problem is alcohol, you don't need AA. Just stop drinking! My problem wasn't alcohol, it was alchol*ism*. After I stopped drinking, I felt worse than when I drank. I didn't use alcohol anymore, but I still had the 'ism.'

"You see," Clancy said, "my life was like the area around Mount St. Helena after the eruption. The volcanic ash covered everything and everything was gray. That's what my life was like. Everything was gray. No color! My job was gray, my wife was gray, my kids were gray, my automobile was gray, my friends were gray—I can't stand a gray life! I need color! And alcohol provided color for me."

This set me to thinking not only about alcoholism but also about several other maladaptations to life. Here's what I came up with.

In medicine we have a number of "deficiency syndromes" that occur when the body lacks an essential nutrient. There is iron deficiency, Vitamin C deficiency, vitamin D deficiency, etc. Each of these conditions has very specific symptoms. Iron-deficiency=anemia. Vitamin C deficiency=easy bruising. Vitamin D deficiency=bone deformity. Doctors know what to look for, what tests to use to confirm the diagnosis, and how to treat these conditions. Obviously, the treatment of any deficiency syndrome is to supply the missing nutrient. Iron deficiency will be cured only by the administration of iron. Even large doses of vitamins will not cure it.

The human being is a composite creature, comprised of a body + something else. Our body is essentially an animal body, and what makes us distinct and unique as human beings is that "something else," which consists of those things that animals do not have.

Allow me to repeat what was said earlier (p.4f) about spirituality. Some of the more obvious uniquely human features, are (1) greater intelligence, (2) the ability to learn from the history of past generations, (3) the ability to reflect on the purpose and goals of life, (4) the ability to volitionally improve oneself, (5) the ability to think about future consequences of one's actions, (6) the ability to defy bodily drives and make moral and ethical choices, etc. I'm sure you can come up with many more traits that people have that are not present in animals in the wild.

I group all these together and say that *the sum total of all the traits that are unique to humans is what we refer to as the "spirit."* As you can see, there are no frankly religious elements in this definition. One can certainly add a religious dimension to it.

If one exercises the elements of the spirit, then one is being *spiritual*. Spirituality can be thought of as being the best human being one can be.

Just as the body requires essential nutrients, so does the spirit. *If we do not provide the spirit with its essential nutrients, we develop a **spirituality deficiency syndrome.***

Just as there are specific symptoms in the physical deficiency syndrome, so also there is a specific symptom of the spirituality deficiency syndrome. That symptom is *discontent*. Discontent is not the same as depression, which is a psychiatric disorder. Discontent is a pervasive, nonspecific feeling of lack of happiness. Discontent is what Clancy referred to as "a gray world."

A gray world may be intolerable for many people. Clancy found relief from the grayness of the world in alcohol. Others find it in drugs, in gambling, in sex, in food, in money or in fame.

We rarely attribute our discontent to lack of spirituality. It is so easy to blame it on other things, and try to change these things in the hope of getting relief from the discontent. One person may blame it on the job and change jobs, on the house and change houses, on the community and move to another city, on the spouse and divorce.

Clancy helped me focus on the "gray world" as depicting the discontent that plagues many people. When he stopped drinking, the grayness of the world returned, and he found sustained relief in pursuit of spirituality, the essential nutrient he had been lacking.

This helped me realize that many therapists are making a serious mistake if they do not discuss spirituality with their clients. While a case may be made for religion being beyond the scope of psychotherapy, the same cannot be said for spirituality as defined here. Failure to identify lack of spirituality as a cause for discontent may result in therapy that is less than adequate.

When spirituality is sought, the discontent begins to dissipate. The need for spirituality as the specific element in the pursuit of happiness is hardly exclusive to the alcoholic. However, it is AA that has recognized this more than anyone else. If we think a bit about spirituality and see what role it plays in our lives, we may be able to do something definitive about our discontent.

We may not appreciate the importance of spirituality until we start working at it. This, too, was a concept I learned from Clancy, as the next anecdote shows.

START ROWING, THE BOAT WILL APPEAR

Clancy was one of the early people to recover through AA. In those days, rehabilitation centers were unheard of. He compared going to a rehabilitation center to a man standing at the banks of a river, when a boat pulls up. "Want to get across the river?" someone says. "Hop in."

"In my days," Clancy said, "there were no rehabilitation centers. It was like someone standing at the river bank, when two guys come along. 'Want to get across the river?' they ask. 'Yes,' the man says. They say, 'O.K. Start rowing.'

"But there is no boat," the man protests.

"Never mind," the two guys say. "Just start rowing. The boat will appear."

"It sounds crazy, but there's nothing else you can do, so you start rowing. And you know what? The boat does appear."

In today's world, there are so many things that are done for us. Thousands of things are ready-made, from fast foods to pre-fab homes. You want French fries? Don't bother peeling and slicing potatoes. Just pick up a bag of pre-cut potatoes and put them into the oven. There are not too many things that we must start from scratch. As a result, when we encounter a task where we must start from scratch, we may be stymied and give up. How can you row when there's no boat? But if you're really determined to get something done, you start anyway, and as you progress, the boat appears.

Think of all the revolutionary inventions. Once a primitive plane flew, it was only a question of further development to produce propeller planes, then jet planes, then super-sonic planes. But what about the Wright brothers? They had nothing to improve upon. All they had was an idea and determination. They started rowing, and the boat appeared. This was equally true of Edison and of all great inventors.

We encounter many challenges in life where we may have nothing but an idea of what we would like. We may even understand the importance of spirituality, and would gladly have it if it could be delivered to our doorstep. Given the prevailing attitude of having so many things "ready for the pot," we may be discouraged when we cannot find spirituality in an easy, "just add water and serve" package. That's when Clancy's teaching kicks in. Begin working toward your goal. Begin working toward spirituality. Start implementing or enhancing the components of spirituality of which I have spoken. Just start rowing, and the boat will appear.

WHEN YOU CAN'T MAKE AMENDS

My home phone is unlisted, but this must be the world's worst kept secret. Inasmuch as I am a rabbi, I get many phone calls from people who think that being both a psychiatrist and a rabbi, I must have the answer to their problems. I am somewhat irritated that after a strenuous day, my evenings at home are interrupted. This is essentially the dispensing of free psychiatric advice. I am especially peeved when people call *collect.* However, I always accept the charges. For all I know, the caller may be on the way to jumping off a bridge, and stopped off at a pay phone in a last desperate attempt to ask for help.

One night, after an especially harrowing day at work which delayed my return home until late, I sat down to dinner at 10 PM. Just as I began eating, the phone rang. My wife had laryngitis and could not answer. I lifted the receiver to hear the operator say, "I have a call for Dr. Twerski." Rather brusquely I said, "Who from?" and I was given a name I did not know. I said "O.K." anyway.

The woman said that she is bi-polar and is on lithium. She has one child and desperately desires more children, but may not conceive while she is taking lithium. "Is there any other way to prevent a relapse if I stop taking lithium?" she asked.

I calmly told her that if she stopped the lithium she was at risk of relapse, but that she should ask her obstetrician to consult with her psychiatrist whether she should take the risk and how best to manage her case. But then I got angry.

"This was not an emergency," I said in a very angry tone. "You could have called me at the office tomorrow instead of at my home late at night. And you have some audacity to call me collect." With that I slammed the receiver down.

I said to my wife, "What gall, to call me collect!" Then it struck me that the operator had not asked whether I would accept the charges. She asked for Dr. Twerski because it was a person-to-person call, but I had assumed it was collect. I felt bad that I had wrongly reprimanded the woman.

I wished I could apologize to her, but I had no idea of her identity. What was I to do? Put an ad in the New York Times: "If you are the person who called Dr. Twerski Wednesday night, I'm sorry I shouted at you?" I felt guilty and there was no way I could make amends to her.

I did not sleep well at all that night. The guilt gnawed at me through the next day. I realized that the only way I could get some relief was to go to an AA meeting.

I shared my feelings at the meeting. One of the group said, "Well, what good is going to come out of eating your heart out? It's not going to make her feel any better." True, but that didn't help much.

Then another person said, "Look, Doc. You feel sorry for how you acted and would really like to apologize, but you can't. Whenever something is out your hands, turn it over to a Higher Power. God will put it in her heart to forgive you."

That made sense. There was no purpose in my trying to do what I couldn't, so let God figure out a way. I felt relieved. With all due respect to my profession, I doubt if any psychiatrist could have helped me the way this man did.

THE TOXICITY OF RESENTMENTS

Andrew's story is not unfamiliar. As a bright corporate attorney he was able to maintain his position in spite of progressively increased drinking. He refused to attend AA meetings because he knew he could do it himself. On his fourth detoxification I prescribed Antabuse (a medication which causes a very severe physical reaction if one ingests any alcohol) and told him that he was to attend meetings daily. If he stopped the Antabuse without my permission or missed even a single AA meeting, I assured him I would have him court-committed to a state hospital. (In 1971 this was an option.)

Andrew attended meetings grudgingly, and after four months actually joined AA. "Just keep coming back," Andrew says. "If you don't get the program, it will get you."

After a year of sobriety, there was a corporate shake-up and Andrew was out. As a result of his drinking he had squandered his earnings and was deeply in debt. A group of investors engaged him to open several retail specialty stores. They formed a corporation and elected Andrew president. When the three stores he opened were operating successfully, the group voted Andrew out. It was clear that they had exploited him.

Andrew was now 37. Never having been in private practice, he had no clients. In order to feed his family, he took on cases which are usually handled by neophytes just getting started.

I ran into Andrew and asked him how he was faring. "I'm very bitter about what they did to me, and I am full of resentments. But I will go to a meeting tonight and try to dump the resentments. You see, if I hang on to resentments, I will drink again."

It occurred to me that Andrew had an insight not shared by too many people. He knew that harboring resentments was destructive, because it would lead him to drink. How many millions of people carry grudges and do not try to divest themselves of them? Perhaps these might not lead them to drink, but smoldering anger can be very destructive. It can cause high blood pressure, heart disease, digestive disorders and migraines. Unlike Andrew, many people are not aware that harboring resentments is toxic.

Anger is a complex feeling. You do not have much choice whether or not to feel angry when you are provoked or offended. That is virtually a reflex reaction. You *do* have a choice about how to react, and you also have a choice about how long to allow the anger to linger.

A person may exercise restraint and not react violently when provoked to anger. However, if the anger lingers, it may lead to unwise judgments and more subtle reactions which are frequently self-destructive.

Some people think that discharging their anger by breaking things or hitting a punching bag will eliminate resentments. This is not true. In fact, such behavior may *reinforce* the anger.

How does AA help one to get rid of resentments? At one meeting I heard someone say, "Harboring resentments is letting someone whom you don't like live inside your head without paying any rent." It occurred to me that he was absolutely correct. The person who is the object of my resentments couldn't care less how I feel about him. My resentments don't bother him a bit. I'm the one who suffers the consequences of the anger eating at my insides. Why should I suffer just because another person acted improperly? It doesn't make any sense.

This is not a complicated, philosophic observation. It can be effective because it is simple. Verbalizing resentments and getting feedback from people who have managed to overcome grudges can be life-saving.

Ecclesiastes had it right. "Anger rests in the bosom of a fool" (7:9). You may not be able to avoid getting angry, but it is most foolish to let it stay with you.

By the way, they say that elephants never forget. If you hurt a dog once, he will remember it. Holding on to a grudge is not uniquely human. That is a trait we share with animals. Getting over resentments is uniquely human, and that makes us more spiritual.

COPING

There may not be too many things in life that we can change, but there are many things about which we can change our attitude.

Anonymous

IT'S GOING TO TURN OUT O.K.

I'm sure you've had days when Murphy's laws were in full swing. Anything that could go wrong, does. These are days when we realize we would have been better off pulling the covers over our heads and staying in bed until 4 PM.

I had a morning like that in Manhattan. Flat tire, stopped by a police officer for driving ten miles above the limit, not finding an open parking lot, and so on. By noon I was fit to be tied. I felt that the only thing that could get me out of the quicksand was an AA meeting. A call to the local AA office produced no less than four meetings within a six block radius.

The speaker was a young woman of thirty-five. She had started drinking at twelve and drugging at fifteen. This led to delinquent, decadent behavior. In spite of suffering the consequences of living on the street, she was a slave to her drug addiction.

At twenty-six she found her way into Alcoholics Anonymous and Narcotics Anonymous, and at the present time was nine years clean and sober.

I had heard similar stories countless times, and this one did little for me. But I have never been to a meeting that I didn't take away something of help. What I took away from this meeting has served me well.

Toward the end of her talk, the woman said, "I must tell you something else before I finish.

"I am a football fan, a rabid Jets fan. I'll never miss watching a Jets game.

"One weekend I had to be away, so I asked a friend to record the game on her VCR. When I returned, she handed me the tape and said, 'By the way, the Jets won.'

"I started watching the tape, and it was just horrible! The Jets were being mauled. At half-time they were behind by twenty points. Under other circumstances, I would have been a nervous wreck. I would have been pacing the floor and hitting the refrigerator. But I was perfectly calm, because I knew they were going to win.

"Ever since I turned my life over to God, I no longer get uptight when things don't go my way. I may be twenty points behind at half time, but I know it's going to turn out o.k. in the end."

Another speaker related a rather typical history of alcoholism, and said, "When I lost my job, I was angry at God. 'Why are You doing this to me? What did I ever do to You to deserve this?' Of course, I didn't see that my drinking had anything to do with my losing my job.

"When my marriage broke up, it was the end of the world for me. There was just nothing else to live for. I don't know what kept me from killing myself."

"A close friend of mine from work was in the program, and I reluctantly went to an AA meeting with her. I didn't have anything else to do. Gradually I took to the program and it has saved my life.

"I can now see how sick my marriage was, and that I never should have been in it. I went back to school and I am now getting my master's degree. This never could have happened had I remained at that job. I can see that this was God taking away from me those things that I did not have the good sense to get rid of by myself. What I thought were terrible tragedies were blessings.

"I can now see a pattern. Anything bad that happens is a prelude to something good. So, when something bad happens I get excited. I can't wait to see what good thing is coming my way."

"I've read about the example of a man who knew nothing about agriculture seeing a farmer sowing seeds. He said, 'How foolish of that man to be taking good grain and burying it in the ground.' He did not know that these seeds would bring a bountiful crop."

Some people at AA have said that "God never shuts a door but that He opens a window." That is not too much of a consolation. A window opening is much smaller than a doorway.

The woman who I quoted did not see it as a window instead of a door. She saw it as burying seeds which will yield a rich crop.

Such women as these have been able to quell their anxiety by their belief that a benevolent God would look after them. Others who do not make the "leap of faith" may nevertheless be able to cope with a challenge if they could reduce its enormity.

We can look back at many things that seemed to be calamities when they occurred. Looking at them years later through a "retrospectoscope", we may indeed see that some of them were actually blessings in disguise, and while others may not have been blessings, they were not the horrific tragedies we thought them to be. The challenges of the present may be so stressful that we may magnify them. Let's remember that we overcame other hurdles in life that appeared gigantic at the time. We can overcome new hurdles, too.

What this young woman said has come to my rescue many times when circumstances are very thorny. I may be twenty points behind at half time, but I can still win.

ACCEPTING A DIFFICULT REALITY

One of the most difficult of psychological problems is unresolved grief. When a person loses a loved one, the emotional pain may be intense. The reaction of grief and the mourning rituals of some religions may enable a person to adjust to the new reality.

It is not unusual for a person in grief to be unable to sleep or eat. The concerned family may consult a physician, who may prescribe sedative or tranquilizing medication. These medications may indeed relieve the distress because they are emotional anesthetics, decreasing the pain of the loss. However, this does not give the mourner the ability to work through the pain, which is a healthy reaction to reality. Anesthetizing the person emotionally is a kind of denial of reality. If the mourner does not accept reality, the grief work may not get done. Some time later, even years later, the person may develop symptoms which are due to delayed and unresolved grief. These symptoms can be very stubborn and treatment may be difficult

A person in grief needs the empathy and support which will enable him to accept and cope with the painful reality. Denial of the reality, with or without medications, is psychologically unhealthy.

Acceptance of reality may be very difficult. Here is an example of a person who achieved acceptance.

At an Al-Anon meeting, a woman related her story. She had just celebrated her thirty-fourth wedding anniversary. The first seventeen years were fraught with the misery of her husband's drinking. The last seventeen years were of recovery.

"After three years of marriage and not having become pregnant," she said, "I made the rounds of specialists. I was finally told to accept that I would never be able to carry a child. That was difficult to accept, but because adoption was an option, I was able to accept it.

"We adopted two lovely children, and after my husband stopped drinking, we had a happy family. When I turned forty, I decided it was time to give up smoking. I went through several weeks of very unpleasant withdrawal.

"After several weeks of feeling good again, the symptoms returned. I consulted my doctor and found out that I was not in nicotine withdrawal at all. I was pregnant! The impossible had occurred. I had been blessed with a miracle.

"I thought that I had rid myself of all bitterness and resentment, but they returned in a crescendo when the nurse put Jimmy in my arms. He was a Down Syndrome child. 'God,' I said, 'why did You do this to me? I had made peace with not having a child of my own. We have a beautiful family with our two adopted children. Why did You deceive me to think I would be happy with a child I carried, and then hit me with this?'

"Every night, my husband and I prayed over the crib. 'God,' we said, 'we know that You can do anything. You have done so many miracles for us. Please, do just one more. Change him.'

"Night after night we prayed for a miracle. Then one day the miracle happened. God changed *us*!"

I felt a chill going up and down my spine. I had never heard the serenity prayer articulated as powerfully as this. (God, grant me the serenity to accept that which I cannot change, the courage to change that which I can and the wisdom to know the difference.) They had been praying for the wrong thing! They wanted to change the unchangeable. But God knew what they really needed, and He gave them the courage to cope with this challenge.

The woman continued, "Now, if this child did not come into the world for anything else other than what I am about to tell you, it would all have been worth it. Because, when I sit in the rocker holding Jimmy in my arms, and I see his short, stubby fingers, and the way his eyes are, you know, and I know how much I love that child with all his shortcomings, that's when I can understand how much God can love me even with all my shortcomings."

I was able to share this with a young couple who had a Down Syndrome child, and they said that it did ease their distress.

Acceptance of reality may be very difficult. Sometimes, even though we cannot find a silver lining to the cloud, we may be able to see how a tragic event may, in some way, be constructive.

I maintained my pulpit throughout medical school and internship. One night, I received a call from a hospital that a woman was requesting a rabbi. When I arrived at the hospital, I found a distressed woman bent over a bassinet. Her child was born with a heart defect that was, in those days (1959) inoperable. Her child was going to die.

The woman looked up at me tearfully and said, "Why, rabbi, why? Nine months of a difficult pregnancy, all for nothing?" I could not answer her question, and I told her that we are not privy to God's secrets. I offered to say a prayer with her.

I left the hospital with a very distressing feeling of being powerless. I was both a rabbi and a physician, and even being armed with the strength of both professions, I could not comfort the woman.

The following morning I told my father how distressed I was. He said to me, "Are you really feeling the mother's pain, or is your distress because your ego has been offended by your feeling of powerlessness? If the latter, then you did not empathize with the woman, because you were too absorbed in your personal distress. Try to overcome your ego problem, then go back and share this woman's pain."

My father continued, "This woman's carrying and delivering the child was not all for naught. This has profoundly affected her emotionally, and it made a change in her. She is not the same person she was before the pregnancy. We cannot understand why God brought about this change in her in so terribly a painful way, but then, we do not have the answer to any suffering."

I went back that day to my internship at my hospital. My delusion of omnipotence, which is not uncommon among physicians, had been shattered. When the day was over, I went back to the woman at the hospital. She appeared pleased to see me. I said, "I don't have an answer to your question, but may I cry with you?" Looking at the infant struggling for air in the oxygenated incubator and at the pain on the mother's face, the tears came readily.

Together with the woman, I recited Psalm 23. She said, "Thank you, rabbi."

The stress of reality difficulties is not resolved by tranquilizers. Sharing the distress with the sufferer does not correct the problem nor eliminate the pain, but may make it just a bit less severe.

In this case, my acceptance of the reality of my powerlessness may have made it just a bit easier for the woman to accept her painful reality.

There are ways in which people try to ease the pain of an unpleasant reality. The next chapter tells of a woman who tried to ease the pain of her reality by making reality *more* painful. Sounds confusing? Read on.

WELCOME DISCOMFORT

In the question and answer period following a lecture to a group of visiting nurses, one nurse said, "There is one elderly woman whom I visit regularly. She is a crotchety old woman who is never satisfied with anything I do. 'You made that blood pressure cuff too tight. It's hurting my arm.' When I sponge bathe her, 'The water is too cold. You're making me shiver.' If I go over the schedule of her medicines, 'You're confusing me. Now I don't know when to take anything.' It's so frustrating! But to top it off, when I leave, she says, 'You're coming back next week, aren't you?' If she doesn't like my service, why does she want me back? She could call the office and request a different nurse."

I was able to solve the problem thanks to something I learned from an octogenarian.

Mrs. Glass had been very active in the ladies auxiliary of my father's congregation. She visited our home frequently, even before I was born. She had watched me grow from my infancy.

When I was an intern, I was called to start an intravenous on Mrs. Glass, who was in her late eighties and was hospitalized because of pneumonia. She had undergone amputation of a leg due to complications of diabetes. She recognized me and we chatted a bit. Then I told her I was going to start her intravenous. "It won't hurt much," I said. "Just a tiny prick of a needle."

Mrs. Glass said, "Foolish child! Let it hurt a lot. Do you think one likes to leave a world that is comfortable?"

It took a bit for Mrs. Glass' words to sink in. What she was saying was that when a person knows his time on earth is running out and he must soon leave it, it is easier if he can see the world as a miserable place. Leaving a pleasant world is much harder.

A perfect vacation is one that had excellent weather for golfing, hiking, swimming and other outdoor activities, then ends up with the last two days being cold, wet and dreary. This makes leaving the vacation resort much easier. If the weather is warm and sunny, it is difficult to leave such a wonderful place to go back to the office.

Mrs. Glass actually wanted to feel that the world was an uncomfortable place. It made the acceptance of the inevitable a bit easier.

The elderly lady who was dissatisfied with everything the nurse did was simply trying to make her departure from the world less painful. She really liked the nurse, as her request "You're coming back, aren't you?" indicated, but in order for her to see the world as a miserable place, she had to complain.

People who care for the elderly are sometimes frustrated by the apparent futility in trying to please them. Mrs. Glass' comment should help them understand that the complaints of these people are not really an expression of dissatisfaction, but a way in which they try to cope with the realization that their time in the world is running out.

The visiting nurse's patient had to fabricate discomfort where none existed, but it is actually possible for a person to be thrilled in having *real* pain. Sounds absurd? I was able to use what I learned to help a young man with his suffering in the following incident.

CAN THERE BE JOY IN HURTING?

A young woman was involved in a terrible automobile accident, sustaining numerous injuries. One of these resulted in the severance of the nerves from the spinal cord to her right arm. As a result, she had no sensation and no motion of the right arm. The surgeons performed a nerve repair, bringing the torn ends of the nerves together. However, this is not like splicing two ends of a torn electric wire, which allows the current to be conducted. In the case of a nerve repair, return of function depends on the growth of the upper part of the nerve through channels in the lower part. If such growth does not occur, the joining of the nerves accomplishes nothing. The young woman was told that it would be several months before the success or failure of the operation was known. Her right arm was put in a sling, and she had to wait to find out whether she would regain the function of her arm.

After several months, the young woman was playing cards, holding the cards in her left hand as well as a cigarette. In trying to manipulate the cards, she dropped the cigarette, which fell on her right hand and she felt the burn. She promptly threw the cards in the air, jumped up, and ran around, jumping up and down for joy and shouting, "It's hurting! It's hurting!" The pain of the burn indicated that her sensation was returning. The surgery had been successful, and she would regain the use of her right arm.

Under other circumstances, a person who sustains a burn might say, "Ouch!" perhaps accompanied by some expletives. For this woman, the discomfort of the pain was obscured by the realization that she would regain the use of her right arm, and the pain was more than welcome.

I was able to use the lesson of this incident at the rehabilitation center. One day, a young man met me in the corridor and asked to speak with me. We stepped into a nearby room, whereupon he threw his arms around me and began sobbing, "You've got to help me, Doc. I can't take it! I can't take it! It's too much pain."

I asked the young man, "When did you come here?"

"Two days ago," he said.
"How old are you?" I asked.
"Twenty-four," he said.
"When did you start using drugs?" I asked.
"At twelve," he answered.
"And since age twelve, what is the longest period of time that you went without using a chemical?" I asked.
"I haven't ever gone without a chemical," he said.
"I want you to listen to this story," I said, and I told him about the woman who was thrilled at feeling the pain of the burn. "Do you understand why she was happy?" I asked. He said, "Yes."

"You are no different," I said. "For the past twelve years, you have anesthetized your system with drugs, so that you were not able to feel anything. You can't live a normal life without feeling. Now the anesthetic effect of the drugs is wearing off, and you feel pain for the first time in twelve years. Your feeling system is returning to normal, and the pain you feel is like the burn this young woman felt. Instead of crying about the pain, you should be jumping for joy like the woman, shouting, 'Hurray! I'm hurting! I'm going to be able to feel again.' With an intact sensory system, you will also be able to feel love, pride and joy.

"We can't take your pain away with a magic wand," I said, "but now that your ability to feel is coming back, we'll help you deal with the feelings."

It is only normal to have a reflex reaction to pain, but we should give more thought to the significance of pain. There may be no redeeming feature of a toothache or stomach ache, but emotional pain may be a harbinger of recovery and growth. Discomfort may be constructive, as in the following episode.

A REFRESHER COURSE

One of my favorite AA meetings was held downtown at noon on Friday. The lunchtime downtown meeting was attended by many business people and lawyers. At one meeting, John, an executive, asked me if I could stay for a few moments after the meeting.

I knew John well. Several years earlier I had said to him, "You've been sober a long time, John, haven't you?" John just shrugged. "Well, how long have you been sober?" I asked.

John pulled a little calendar from his pocket, turned the pages and said, "9,842 days."

"How many years is that?" I asked.

John responded, "I don't know, Doctor. Yesterday was 9,842 days. If I make it through today by the grace of God, it'll be 9,843 days." John took "one day at a time" very seriously.

After the meeting, John said to me, "I'm having a bad day, Doctor. I haven't had a day like this in thirty-three years."

"You mean you feel like drinking today?" I asked. John nodded affirmatively. "I can't understand it. I feel depressed, and I'm craving a drink to feel better."

"Wonderful!" I exclaimed. "That's great!"

John looked at me quizzically. "Why do you say that?"

I said, "John, how many times have I asked you to recommend someone who could 12-step (provide help for sobriety) a newcomer?"

"Lots of times," John said.

"And how many times have I asked you to 12-step someone yourself?" I asked.

"You never have," John admitted.

"Haven't you ever wondered why? You see, John, when I have someone who needs 12-stepping, he's a person who is just hours or days away from his last drink. He is struggling, in agony. He needs to know how to get through this suffering without taking a drink. What can you do for him? Tell him like it was thirty-three years ago? What good does that do? He might as well read it in a book."

"A newcomer needs someone who can identify and empathize with him. You are so far away from your last drink that you are not struggling anymore. You can't be of much help to a newcomer. That's why I haven't asked you to 12-step anyone."

"But today things are changing. You're uncomfortable and you're fighting the urge to drink. I suggest that you go to a beginner's meeting tonight."

The next day John called me. He was feeling much better, and had gone to a beginner's meeting.

"That's good," I said. "Now will you please go up to room 616 in the hospital and talk to the patient there? You can help him."

John told me that after this incident, his talks at AA meetings had taken on a new freshness. "My talks had become stale because my recovery was stale. You were right, Doctor. That bad day was a blessing."

In AA and out of AA, struggle and challenge are stimuli for growth. Every period of distress can be a new opportunity for growth.

The night before John died at age eighty-three, he entered into his calendar, 16,177 days. One day at a time.

Although John had been sober for many years prior to this "bad day," he was able to achieve additional spiritual growth.

The close association of discomfort with growth was not apparent to me until I discovered something about lobsters.

THE PAIN OF LEARNING

At one AA meeting, the speaker related the misery he had experienced during his active addiction. Then he challenged the audience with a question. "Can anyone tell me anything they have ever learned from a pleasurable experience?"

I had never thought of it quite that way. I could not think of anything I had learned from a really enjoyable experience, other than to try to repeat it.

If I had designed the world, I would have made all learning painless. But I did not design the world and God did. For reasons known only to Him, He made much learning painful. That is reality and we must accept it.

I must repeat what I read in a magazine in a dentist's waiting room. The article was headed, "How Do Lobsters Grow?" Come to think of it, how *can* a lobster grow? It is encased in a rigid, hard shell which does not expand.

The answer is that when the lobster grows, the shell becomes confining and oppressive. The lobster then retreats under a rock to be safe from predatory fish, sheds the shell, and produces a more spacious one. As the lobster continues to grow, the new shell eventually becomes oppressive, and the lobster will repeat the process of shedding the confining shell and producing a larger shell. This process is repeated until it has reached its maximum growth.

So much for the article. Interesting, huh? But don't overlook the crucial point. The signal the lobster has that it's time to shed the shell is -- *discomfort*! If lobsters had access to doctors, they might never grow. Why? Because when they felt the discomfort of the oppressive shell, they would get a prescription for a pain-killer or a tranquilizer. With the discomfort gone, they would not shed the shell and produce a more spacious one. They would die as tiny little lobsters.

For human beings too, discomfort is often a signal that it's time to grow.

There are indeed bona-fide depressive illnesses and other psychiatric conditions that may require anti-depressant medication. But the largest classification of drugs bought in the U.S, is the *tranquilizers*, the powdered equivalent of alcohol, to which so many people resort, because they are uncomfortable rather than because they have a psychiatric illness.

The speaker was right. Much of emotional pain is nature's way of telling us that it's time to grow. How foolish to take chemicals which eliminate the stimulus that can make us better human beings!

Remember the "Spirituality Deficiency Syndrome?" The discontent is nature's way of telling us that we have not fulfilled ourselves as human beings. Instead of anesthetizing ourselves or finding scapegoats for our discontent, we should pursue happiness by growth in character.

NOTHING TO FEAR BUT FEAR

At one meeting the speaker said, "I was always plagued by fear. Sometimes I didn't know what I was afraid of, so I conjured up things which I could think of as frightening. I think all alcoholics live in constant fear."

I was driving to a spirituality retreat with a friend in recovery, and we were listening to an audio-tape of an AA speaker who said, "I always felt like I was walking through a mine-field, where the next step I take might blow me to bits. If the next step turns out to be safe, it may be the one after that that will destroy me."

My friend hit the brakes and pulled the car off onto the shoulder of the road. He was visibly shaken. "That's how I felt," he said. "I can't believe that anyone else felt like that."

Many alcoholics have said that the one trait common to all alcoholics is fear. This fear sometimes manifests itself as morbid expectations.

Bob told about his elation when he became sober. He was sure that he would never drink again. Three days before his first anniversary of sobriety, Bob got drunk.

"Please believe me," he said, "this was not like before. I really did not want to drink, and I didn't have the craving.

"Everything was going good for me. Too good. I was never so happy before. I was doing so well at my job that I got a promotion. For the first time I can remember, my wife told me how much she loved me. It was unbelievable. Now I was approaching a year of sobriety. I hadn't been sober for even one week since age twelve. This was too good to be true. I felt I didn't deserve this happiness and that something terrible was going to happen. Every time the phone rang, I panicked. It's going to be a call to tell me that my little girl was hit by a car. I couldn't take the tension of the impending disaster that I expected to happen. So I drank to break the jinx. I didn't enjoy the drinking the way I used to. In fact, I hated it. But I had to do it to ward off any other disaster."

I understood Bob. Morbid expectations are not unique to alcoholics. Non-alcoholics often experience them, unless they can be helped by a psychologist. But most people don't seek psychological help, and although they may not resort to drink, they may do other things that may be as destructive as what Bob did.

In addition to psychotherapy, sharing these thoughts with a trusted friend may help. Unfortunately, because we may realize that these thoughts are groundless, we may be reluctant to reveal them to anyone else. Here, recovering alcoholics have an advantage. They verbalize these fears at meeting, and sharing them with other people may help a person recognize how irrational they are. Discovering that one is not unique in having such feelings can also provide some relief.

WHY CRY WHEN YOU CAN LAUGH?

Some newcomers, upon entering an AA meeting for the first time, say, "I must be in the wrong place. If all these people are sober, how come they seem so happy? How come they're laughing? I haven't had a drink for a week and I'm downright miserable. I don't feel a bit like laughing."

That's just one of the wonderful things about AA. Think about it for a moment. Something happened in the past that was very upsetting to you. If you cry about it, how much good will that do? You might as well laugh about it. Laughter is very therapeutic.

Obviously, there are unfortunate occurrences that we can never laugh about and that will always evoke tears. But there are also things that we can laugh about, although they may have been unpleasant at the time they occurred.

In AA meetings people tell about their past and they laugh about themselves. Everybody shares and laughs *with* them. No one laughs *at* them.

Some of the stories about their antics are indeed very funny. One of the funniest was not about what they did while drinking, but while in recovery.

Edgar said that after five years of sobriety, he had not done a Fifth Step, which requires "admitting to another human being the exact nature of our wrongs." "The kinds of things I did when I was drunk are so disgusting," he said, "that I could never again face the person who knew. So I didn't tell anyone.

"The firm I was working for did business with a company in South Africa, and they sent me to Johannesburg to negotiate a contract. Of course, I looked up AA in Johannesburg and went to a meeting. I exchanged greetings with the man next to me, and told him I was from the U.S. on business.

"I suddenly had a bright idea. Here was man I would never run into again. I told him I needed to talk to someone, and he invited me to his home after the meeting. I then unloaded everything I had been keeping bottled up for many years. I left his home at 2:30 AM feeling that a heavy burden had been lifted. I was ecstatic.

"The next day I met with my counterpart. After we finished all the minutiae of the contract, he said, 'I am authorized to sign contracts up to $250,000. This contract is for over $600,000, so it will require the signature of the CEO. It's just a formality and won't take more than a few minutes.'

"I accompanied him to the CEO's office, and O! My God! This was the man to whom I had revealed my worst secrets last night! I almost died!

"The CEO smiled, quickly glanced over the contract and signed it.

"I had traveled 8,000 miles to do my Fifth Step with someone whom I knew I would never meet again!"

We all laughed along *with* Edgar.

What did I take away from that meeting besides having a good laugh? I guess it taught me that there is no way to outsmart God. If He wanted Edgar to be able to face someone to whom he had revealed everything about himself, He arranged it.

Can laughter be helpful in coping? Sometimes. When something upsetting to you occurs, just think, "Five years from now, when I look back at this incident, am I going to be able to laugh about it? Don't I laugh now at some things that I thought were terrible five years ago? Well, if I'm going to laugh about it later, why not laugh about it now?"

Children don't wait five years. They cry bitterly when they scrape their knees. But five *minutes* later, they may be rollicking and having a good time.

This is something we can learn from children.

GRATITUDE

One of the most frequent words at AA meetings is "grateful." Almost every speaker will say, "I am grateful for my recovery," or "I am grateful that I was given a second chance." Sometimes a person will say, "I am grateful for being alcoholic. My life was crazy even before I drank. I never would have straightened it out if I had not gotten into the program. Sure, alcohol was my downfall, but it's like tearing down a small building to build a skyscraper in its place."

I always thought of myself as being a grateful person. I appreciated what others did for me and I sincerely thanked them. But there was still something about gratitude that I had to learn.

I had just bought a new car, loaded with everything, especially cruise control. I have a tendency to speed, and I could be speeding without being aware of it. So I use cruise control. For me, that's like Antabuse for the alcoholic. That's the medication I mentioned earlier that makes you deathly ill if you drink, so it gives you the control you don't have.

Well, my cruise control was not accurate. I would set it at 60 mph and it would vacillate between 55 and 65. I could have it fine tuned, but that would mean taking the car to the dealer, spending several hours waiting, etc.

I took my frustration to a meeting. The speaker was a woman who was telling about the wonderful things that had happened to her since she stopped drinking. She has a full time job, and has moved to better quarters for herself and her son. She hopes soon to have enough money to repair her car which needs a new transmission. The reverse gear does not work, so she has to plan her parking to be able to get out of a parking space without going in reverse. When the audience laughed, she said, "Well, I must remember that some people don't have a car at all."

If I could have dug a deep hole in the ground, I would have jumped in. This woman was grateful that she had a car, albeit without a reverse gear, and here I was griping because my fully loaded new car had a cruise control that lacked precision.

I came to the meeting frustrated with the car. I left the meeting frustrated with myself for being an ingrate. I had learned something valuable about gratitude.

GOD NEVER DESERTS

It was one of those days when I awoke in the morning feeling down, for no identifiable reason. In the afternoon, I was standing in front of my house watering the lawn when a car pulled up to the curb and two men jumped out. They were alumni of Gateway Rehabilitation Center.

"Hi, Doc," one said. "How ya doin'?"

"If you guys were not in the program, I would say 'Just fine.' But I don't lie to people in the program. I've had a lousy day."

"You need a meeting, Doc," they said.

"No, thank you," I said. "I'll be all right."

That night the doorbell rang. It was those two guys. "We're here to take you to a meeting," they said.

Just my luck to end up at a "gratitude meeting." Everyone who spoke gave a brief account of how much happier they are in their sobriety. When you feel depressed, the last thing you need is to hear how happy other people are. I sat patiently through the meeting, hoping it would soon be over.

The last speaker said, "I am four years sober, and I wish I could say that they have been good years. My company down-sized and I was let go. I have been unable to find a job. My marriage was on shaky grounds anyway, and this was the clincher. My wife divorced me and got custody of the children."

"My house was foreclosed because I was unable to make the mortgage payments. Last week the finance company repossessed my car. But I can't believe that God brought me all this way just to walk out on me now."

I knew then why I was at that meeting. I have never yet walked away from a meeting without taking something valuable along with me. This meeting served as an effective antidepressant.

In the prayerbook there is a verse, "Your mercies have supported me until now, and I know that You will never abandon me." I had been reciting that prayer regularly for over forty years, but I had never before felt it the way I did after this meeting.

We are often confronted with challenges, some of which may appear to be overwhelming. If we reflect a bit, we will recall that we have weathered challenges in the past that we had thought were overwhelming, and yet we survived. That thought should give us some courage and confidence to cope with what is happening now.

LET GO AND LET GOD

This AA principle is one of the most difficult things for beginners in the recovery program to accept. "What do you mean, 'Let go?'" It is difficult only because they still are under the delusion that they *can* control everything in their lives. Why relinquish control?

Early on in my involvement in AA, I was privileged to get an understanding of this. We were sitting around a table, and a newcomer to the program was expressing his disagreement with "letting go." A veteran in the program remarked, "Okay, so *don't* let go. Now what are you going to do?" The newcomer was baffled, looking for words to respond, and was visibly frustrated. The veteran said, "Look, son, if there is really something you can do, then don't let go. It's just that if you realize that there are things you can't do anything about, it makes no sense to try and do something when there's nothing you can do. That's when you have to let go. Stop wasting your energy. But you first have to realize that you really can't control everything."

The wisdom of these words became evident one day when I was driving down a steep hill on a winter day, assuming the road was dry. It wasn't. It was frozen over and I lost control of the car. The brakes would not hold, and I tried to steer into the curb to stop my descent, but the wheels would not go where I wanted them to. At the bottom of the hill was a busy thoroughfare, and I knew I was going to be killed. If I had been able to think clearly, I would have opened the door and jumped out. I might have broken a couple of limbs, but I would live. If I descended into the busy thoroughfare I would surely be killed. God spared me, and I miraculously crossed the intersection without being hit.

But you can't count on miracles. Logically, I should have jumped out of the car to save my life. Why didn't I jump out? Because I was too busy frantically pumping the brakes and turning the steering wheel, both of which were futile. *I was trying to control the uncontrollable*, and if God hadn't intervened, I would have been killed.

I later realized that we may often fail to see that we are out of control, and we may be so engaged in the futility of trying to control the uncontrollable that we don't do what may be effective. That's where the wisdom of "letting go" comes in.

"Keep it simple." What could be simpler than "Stop trying to do the impossible?"

MANY WORRIES? BE HAPPY!

Like every other person, I do not like to be laden with worries. And, like every other person, I usually have enough of them.

When my brother was seriously ill with cancer, I asked a rabbi friend of mine to keep him in his prayers. This white-bearded sage was a kind man who was very wise. I was, therefore, completely taken aback when, on parting, he said to me, "May you be blessed with many worries."

Noting my bewildered expression at this strange blessing, he explained, "It is impossible for a human being to be totally free of worry. Ever since Adam and Eve were expelled from the Garden of Eden, man has been subject to worry.

"Sometimes a person has something so serious on his mind that it obliterates all other concerns. For example, you are so worried about your brother's illness that it occupies your entire mind, and you do not pay attention to the myriad of other things in your life.

"When a person has only one worry, that is bad. It means that there is something so terribly distressing bothering him that he doesn't think of anything else. If one has many worries, that means that there is nothing so overwhelmingly bad that it obscures everything else.

"It is not realistic to be without any worry. That just does not happen. And it is very bad if a person has only one worry. The best situation, therefore, is for a person to have many worries. That means that there is nothing terribly disturbing going on in one's life.

"My blessing to you was that you should have many worries. That means that nothing really bad is on your mind."

Now when I find I am worried about half a dozen things, I am happy. I even have a different perspective on annoyances, as the next piece explains.

SOME ANNOYANCES ARE GOOD FOR YOU

As a psychiatrist, I am constantly besieged with people's problems. Many of these do indeed require relief. However, sometimes people complain of annoyances which are part of normal life.

As the beneficiaries of modern science and technology, we have eliminated so many of the discomforts that bothered our ancestors, that we have come to believe that life should be free of *all* distress. I think that this view of life is a contributing factor to the serious problem of addiction and chemical dependency that is probably the nation's number one health problem. In addition to illicit drugs, far too many people are escaping from the discomforts of reality into alcohol and tranquilizers. We have lost sight of the fact that some annoyances may actually be beneficial.

A friend of mind had a farm with many fruit trees. His wife had a phobia of bees, and was afraid to go outdoors in the summer for fear of being stung by a bee. To help his wife, my friend used insecticides to get rid of the bees.

The following spring, his fruit trees were covered with beautiful blossoms. Alas! The trees bore no fruit. It was the bees that carried the pollen from blossom to blossom, fertilizing them to develop into fruit. In the absence of bees, there was no fruit.

Were the bees pesky? Yes. But you must make your choice: bees and fruit vs. no bees and no fruit.

Some parents love their children so dearly that they try to protect them from any and all annoyances. That is not very good training for living in the real world. We should show our children how to cope with annoyances rather than eliminate all of them. A life completely free of annoyances may not bear much fruit, like trees without bees.

WE KNOW WHOM WE CAN TRUST

We want to have faith. We need to have faith, but sometimes we may find our faith under stress.

After the attack at the World Trade Center, people gathered in churches, synagogues and mosques to pray. One person interviewed by a television reporter said, "What am I to do? Pray to God to care for the souls of those who were killed? If there is a God who is all powerful, why did He let all those people get killed in the first place?"

This question has been repeatedly asked whenever there is a disaster, whether man-made like the terrorist attack, or a tornado, earthquake or tsunami that causes loss of many lives. No one has any logical answer to this question. The faithful can say only that these are things that are beyond our understanding.

Although I am as incapable of understanding the Divine mysteries as anyone else, I did gain a bit of insight from something I observed in a pediatrician's office.

A mother was sitting with her one-year-old child, who was playing happily with some toys. The doctor, clad in his white coat entered the waiting room. The baby took one look at the doctor and emitted a sharp scream, clinging to his mother for dear life. The baby remembered only too well what this meant. The man with the white coat is a villain, an evil monster who jabs babies with a sharp needle and makes them hurt and sick for two days.

As the mother carried the baby into the treatment room, the baby cried bitterly and struggled against its mother, biting and kicking her. The mother restrained the baby so that the doctor could administer the immunizing injection. As soon as the doctor withdrew the needle and left, the baby threw its arms around the mother's neck, clutching tightly.

As I observed this, I wondered why the baby was holding on to his mother for protection. Wasn't she the one who had just collaborated with the villain to let him hurt him? Hadn't she betrayed him? The baby had no way of knowing that the injection would protect him from terrible diseases. The only answer can be that notwithstanding the fact that she was responsible for his getting hurt, the baby knew that she was nevertheless his protector and the one who cared most for him. There was no way he could understand her uncharacteristic behavior, but this did not detract from his trust in her.

The gap between the infant's intellect and his mother's intellect is indeed vast, but the gap between our intellect and the infinite wisdom of God is unfathomable. Although like the infant, we cannot understand why He allows us to be hurt, our trust in Him is unshakeable.

Whenever I feel like questioning God, I am reminded of the scene in the pediatrician's office. Although I cannot understand, it helps me understand why I cannot understand.

USE AND DISCARD

This insight came to me the first time I saw a "disposable camera."

We have learned about the various eras in human history. There was the Stone Age, the Iron Age, the Bronze Age, etc. I have often wondered, if humanity does survive, what will our era be called? One of the possibilities is that it will be known as "the Disposable Age." Ours is an era in which many things are disposable. Just think of it: disposable gloves, disposable dishes and tableware, disposable tablecloths, disposable slippers, disposable gowns, and more recently disposable contact lenses and now disposable cameras.

When I became Bar-Mitzvah, one of the gifts I received was a Sheaffer fountain pen. I kept it for seventeen years, and when I lost it, I felt the loss. I had become attached to it. Today I rarely buy a pen, because I get complimentary pens at hotels and in a number of promotions. I rarely end up the week with the same ball-point I had at the beginning of the week. When anyone borrowed my Sheaffer pen, I held on to the top to make sure it would be returned. Today, if someone borrows my pen, I don't expect or care to get it back.

I recall being able to take a radio to the repair shop. Now, you would be hard-pressed to find anyone who can repair a radio or tape-recorder. If it breaks, you throw it away and get a new one. Why bother trying to fix it? When my food-processor broke, the appliance repair person told me that it would be cheaper to buy a new one than to repair the old. Even some high-priced items have no durability. Some people will trade in a perfectly functioning automobile every three years. Why? Because! Enough of this old model. A new one will be better.

Don't underestimate the impact of this on our thoughts and emotions. We have developed an attitude that if anything goes wrong with something, don't try to fix it. Just throw it away and get a new one.

Unfortunately, this attitude has carried over to human relationships, and particularly to marriage. Something wrong with the marriage? Don't exert yourself trying to repair it. Get rid of the old spouse and get a new one.

We are not going to deprive ourselves of the conveniences of disposable items, but we should be on our guard that we do not allow the Disposable Age philosophy to affect our personal lives.

EVEN A BAD FALL IS JUST A FALL

In treating alcoholics, it is not unusual for a person to relapse into drinking after a period of abstinence. People sometimes say to him, "You're back to square one. You've got to start from the beginning."

Periods of success followed by a failure are not unique to alcoholism. A person may be successful in business for years, then have a reversal. A student may have excelled in school and then have had a bad semester.

I achieved a perspective on this one winter day when my car would not start, so I walked six blocks to the post office. The streets were a bit icy, so I tried to walk carefully. In spite of my caution, I slipped and fell when I was halfway to the post office. I was bruised, but no broken bones.

Anyone who would have said that because I slipped and fell I was back at my home would have been wrong. I had made three blocks of progress, and that was undeniable. I was much more cautious the rest of the way.

If a person relapses into drinking after a period of sobriety, he is not back to square one. The progress he made during that period cannot be denied. If a youngster fails sixth grade, that does not put him back to kindergarten.

This is equally true of other mishaps. We make mistakes and we learn from them. I have heard it said, "Experience is a hard teacher, but fools will learn no other way." That is wrong. Fools do *not* learn from experience, and they may repeat the same mistake many times. It is the *wise* that learn from experience.

There is an aphorism, "If you fall, look around you. You may see something at ground level that you could not have seen from above." Now *that* is a wise saying.

I am bothered by the fact that after seventy-four years of life and many, many experiences, I still have to learn from mistakes. I thought I should be able to avoid mistakes by now. But inasmuch as I always want to learn, I must make peace with the fact that our best learning is often the result of a mistake. Rather than brood endlessly about having made a mistake, we should value it as a very effective lesson.

STAY WITHIN REALITY

Miracles do happen. However, we should not count on miracles. We should indeed aspire, but our aspirations should not be absurd. Aspiration is a great motivator only when it is reasonable. Even our prayers and wishes should be within the boundaries of reality. It is reasonable, if one so wishes, to pray to win the lottery. True, the chances of winning may be one out of ten million, but someone *does* win, and I may pray that I be that someone. However, the Talmud says, if your wife is pregnant, don't pray that she have a boy or girl. Whatever gender the fetus is has already been decided. God is not going to change the gender, so it is futile to pray for it.

Some people who consult a psychiatrist seem to have no aspirations at all. Others have aspirations that are so far out that they are not achievable. I learned the importance of keeping our aspirations and wishes within the bounds of reality from the cartoon strip, Calvin and Hobbes.

Calvin says to Hobbes, "If you could have a wish, what would you wish for?"

Hobbes says, "I'd wish for a sandwich. I'm hungry."

"Is that all you can wish for?" Calvin asks. "Why, I'd wish for a million, gazillion dollars and my own space shuttle, my private continent, three horses and a fancy sports car.

A bit later they meet again. Hobbes is eating a sandwich. "I got my wish," he said.

Hobbes' wish was well within reality, so he got it. Calvin's wish was so absurd that he got nothing.

As children, we may have the wildest wishes and aspirations. As we mature, our thinking should become more reality oriented so that although we may aim high, our goal should still be within reach. If we retain our juvenile wishes, they are bound to be frustrated, and we may be so disappointed that we may end up losing all aspiration.

We can achieve much in life if we keep our aspirations within reality.

FROM HORSES AND SALMON

You will recall that in the introduction I told you about a rabbi who found deep meaning when he saw several horses with wagons full of hay. I have never been privileged to learn anything from observing horses, but I did learn something from salmon.

I was in a fishery on the west coast and had the opportunity to observe salmon. These fish swim in the Pacific ocean, then they swim upstream, against the tide, to lay their eggs at the place where they were born. It obviously takes much effort to swim against the flow, but they do it. When they encounter a cascade, they jump up against the waterfall. If they don't succeed at making the jump, they swim around a bit to restore their energy, and they try again and again until they succeed. If there are two small cascades together, they never try to jump over both at one time.

I was deeply affected by this. The salmon may not be intelligent. Their drive to get to their spawning place is instinctual, but "knowing" where they must go, they swim against the current to get there. Nothing stops them. If they fail to make a jump, they try again, but they take only one step at a time.

Humans do not have a goal by instinct. We arrive at the knowledge of our goal by means of our intellect. However, once we determine what our ultimate goal is, there should be no obstacle that can stop us. We may have to go against the popular current to achieve our goal, but if we do not succeed, we should not give up. We should keep on trying until we make it. And we should not take a greater bite than we can handle. We should make gradual progress, doing only what is realistically achievable. That's how we can reach our ultimate goal.

Did you know that salmon are good teachers?

THERAPEUTIC TECHNIQUES

HOW TO LISTEN

Good psychotherapists listen to their patients. But listening does not mean just hearing the words they say. Psychotherapeutic listening means sharing the patient's feelings and identifying with the patient.

Of course, there's the story of the young psychiatrist who was totally exhausted at the end of the day. His collar was wilted and his eyes were half closed. On the way out of his office he bumped into a psychiatrist who had his office in the same building. This was a veteran psychiatrist who had been in practice forty years, and who looked fresh as a daisy.

"What's your secret?" the young psychiatrist asked. "How can you keep yourself so spry at the end of the day? I spend the day listening to patients, listening to families, listening to social workers, listening to nurses who call me from the hospital, listening to lawyers involved with my patients. It wears me down. What's your secret?"

The veteran psychiatrist shrugged. "Who listens?" he said.

Good psychotherapists *do* listen. But empathizing with the patient may also compromise the objectivity that is so essential for therapy.

While I did learn much about therapy in my psychiatric training, I learned most about the listening aspect of therapy from my father. He related a story about his great uncle, the chassidic rabbi of Talna.

One morning, after receiving his supplicants for several hours, the rabbi's aide noticed that his clothes were drenched with perspiration. He asked the rabbi, "Why are you perspiring so profusely? You were not doing any physical work."

The rabbi responded, "I wasn't doing any work, you say? Look, when someone comes to me with a problem and I want to help him, I must first feel his problem. That means that I must take my clothes off and put on his clothes. But once I have identified with him, I cannot be of help because I am in his predicament. To extricate myself, I must take off his clothes and put my clothes on again, so that I can be objective. For several hours I've been taking off my clothes and putting on my clothes, taking off my clothes and putting on my clothes, and you say I haven't been doing any work?"

That is where I learned the technique of good therapy. Becoming too involved emotionally in the patient's problem renders the therapist vulnerable to all the distorted feelings that the patient has. Standing aloof as a totally objective observer may make one indifferent to the patient's plight. A therapist must be able to identify and detach, identify and detach. Failure to do both limits the effectiveness of therapy.

A SIMPLE FORMULA

Much of the two years after I completed my psychiatric training was spent in preparing for the National Board exams. Psychiatrists seeking the prestige of "Board Certification" are put through two days of grueling testing on a whole range of subjects in psychiatry and neurology. There is much apprehension that the examiners will ask questions one may not be able to answer, and failing the test is humiliating. Candidates for board certification are understandably anxious. When we assembled for the test, the psychiatrist in charge of the exam said, "I'm going to tell you now what you tell your patients when they are still anxiety-ridden after many months of therapy. You say, 'For heavens sake, pull yourself together.'"

One of the examiners was a psychiatrist with many years of practice behind him. He quizzed me thoroughly, and when he was satisfied that I knew the material, he said, "Son, you know it all just as I did when I was your age. Now I'm going to tell you a simple rule to follow that they did not tell you in training.

"When I was a medical student," he said, "I was fresh out of anatomy, and I observed an operation. I said to the surgeon, 'Is that muscle the *transversus abdominus*?' The surgeon, who had been performing operations for forty years, looked up at me and said, 'It's good for you to know the names of all the muscles when you're in medical school, but when you're doing surgery, just sew the red to the red and the white to the white, and you'll do fine.'

"I want to give you a simple rule to go by in psychiatry. As you know, there's a lot of ideas that get shoved into the subconscious portion of the mind because they are too much for us to handle in our awareness, so we repress them. These are ideas that we're frightened of having. But these ideas don't just lie there in the subconscious. They constantly want to burst into our awareness, so we try to keep them down there. Most people have good enough defenses to keep the lid on.

"Think of it this way. There's a jack-in-the-box sitting on a coiled spring, and it is held down by the lid. If the lid is loose, the jack-in-the-box may pop out. You can put something on the lid to keep it down. If you put too heavy an object on the lid, you may crush it.

"The ideas in the subconscious are like a jack-in-the-box. They want to pop out. If the ego-lid is loose, some crazy ideas will emerge, which can make a person psychotic. If a person is too frightened that unacceptable ideas might emerge into awareness, he may pile on multiple defense mechanisms to keep the ego-lid on. This makes him neurotic.

"Just listen to the patient. If ideas that should be in the subconscious are coming out, try and help the patient repress them and push them back in. If it seems that the patient has piled on too many defenses on the ego-lid, help him lift some of these defenses, leaving just enough to keep the ego-lid on.

"Like the surgeon said to me, follow this rule and you'll do just fine."

I wish someone had taught me this simple rule early in my training. I had one patient who had some ideas emerging in a dream from the subconscious for which repression had failed. I should have said, "Many people have strange thoughts such as these in dreams. It must have been something you ate for dinner that you didn't digest well. Just forget them. They don't mean a thing." Instead, like a scientific psychiatrist, I interpreted the dream material for her. This was a terrible mistake. She could not handle these ideas, and she became psychotic.

When I began teaching first-year residents, the first thing I told them was the rule given to me by the veteran psychiatrist. "If the lid is open, push it down. If it's pressed down too hard, ease the pressure on it." Hopefully, they would not repeat my mistake.

TRANSFERENCE AND COUNTER-TRANSFERENCE

It is not as easy for a psychotherapist to maintain objectivity as, say, an internal medicine physician. A doctor who is not diabetic can be totally objective in treating a diabetic patient. Whatever is going on with the patient does not affect him personally. If the doctor is free of cancer, he can be totally objective in treating a cancer patient. There is a *qualitative* difference between the doctor and the patient.

This is not so in psychotherapy. Every normal human being has had moments of anxiety and depression. The psychotherapist may have some personal difficulties within his own family. The patient may have a problem relating to his in-laws, and if the therapist happens to have in-law problems, investigating this area of the patient's life may cause discomfort for the therapist. To avoid this discomfort, the therapist may shift the focus to other areas of the patient's life, thereby failing to help the patient with this particular problem

In psychotherapy, there is the concept of "transference," which means that the patient brings in attitudes that he has toward others—parents, siblings, spouse, children, boss – and "transfers" them to the therapist, behaving toward the therapist as if he were one of the above. By recognizing this, the therapist can help the patient identify these feelings and correct his distortions of them or help him see how he has allowed these feelings to inappropriately affect other relationships.

Then there is "counter-transference." The therapist, too, is a human being with a variety of attitudes he has developed toward others, and he may transfer these onto the patient.

How can a therapist avoid these pitfalls? I found the answer, in all places, in a book of jokes!

There was a bookkeeper who was a perfectionist. In 35 years, he had never missed a single day's work and had never come to work late. He was meticulous, and his work was always precise to the penny.

He had one habit that was a mystery. When he came to work in the morning, he would unlock his desk drawer, open it, nod knowingly, close the drawer and get to his books. No one bothered to ask him what this daily ritual was all about.

After 35 years of faithful work, he retired. The very next day, all his fellow employees gathered to solve the mystery of the ritual that went on every day for 35 years.

When they opened the drawer, it was empty except for a card that read, "**The debit column is the one facing the window.**"

I emulated the bookkeeper. If you open my desk drawer, you will find a card that says, "**The patient is the one on the other side of the desk.**"

I frequently open the desk drawer to remind me that yes, I may have moments of anxiety or depression, and I may have difficulties in some relationships, but I am functioning well, and the patient's problems in areas similar to mine do not have to trigger a defensive reaction in me.

WHAT A PLUMBER TAUGHT ME

One day at the rehabilitation center, a therapist requested that I see one of his clients. "This fellow has been here for over two weeks," he said, "and he shows no signs of emotion at all. I wonder if he may have a psychiatric problem in addition to his addiction."

The young man was twenty-eight. He was very cooperative in the interview, but in discussing subjects in which some expression of emotion, any emotion, would be normal, there was nothing at all. Among the things he told me was that his father died suddenly when he was ten years old. "I didn't cry. I looked at myself in the mirror and said 'You're not going to cry.'" In this interview, I did not see any sign of any specific psychiatric condition.

The next day, my wife told me that the faucet in the laundry sink was dripping. I am sufficiently handy to be able to change a washer, but to do so, I needed to turn off the water supply to the faucet. However, the valve was stuck, and I was afraid that if I became more aggressive, I might break a pipe and flood the basement. There was no choice but to call a plumber.

But the plumber had no better luck than I did. He said, "This valve is frozen. It has probably never been turned since the house was built seventy-five years ago. The only thing I can do is shut off the main valve, but that will turn off the water supply to the entire house. It shouldn't be for more than fifteen minutes."

A bit later the plumber came up holding the faucet. "You've got a problem, Doc," he said. "It's not the washer. The inside of the faucet is eroded. I'll have to replace the faucet."

"O.K.," I said. "There's not much choice."

"I have to go back to the shop to pick up a faucet," he said. "Your water will be off in the whole house for about two hours."

After the new faucet was installed and the main valve turned back on, the plumber opened the faucet, and a gush of rusty water came out with a frightening explosive force and a loud noise. The plumber explained, "When the main valve was turned off, some air got in the pipes. The first time you open any faucet or shower or flush the toilet, you'll get an explosive discharge of water, but after that it'll be o.k."

It suddenly became clear to me what had happened with the young man. At age ten, he had wanted to protect himself from the painful grief of his father's death. He did not know how to block the isolated emotion of grief, so he did what the plumber did. He shut off the "main valve," turning off *all* emotion. He could feel nothing. After being devoid of feelings for eighteen years, he was afraid to feel anything, even pleasurable emotions. To allow himself now to feel *any* emotion, he would have to turn on the "main valve," but this might result in the emotion coming out with an explosive force that he felt he could not handle. Allowing himself to feel *any* emotion was too threatening, so he kept the "main valve" closed.

Once the problem was identified, we were able to help the young man, offering much reassurance and support to allow him to open his feeling system.

This insight has been very helpful to me. There are many people who seem to be devoid of emotion. This may be because of some occurrence that caused them to turn off their feeling system.

I learned much from this plumber.

TO TELL THE TRUTH

I was privileged to receive a very important personal teaching which has profoundly affected my life style as well as my therapeutic technique. I had a patient who was a chronic complainer, coming up with new physical symptoms frequently. I felt that his complaints were nothing but malingering, an effort to get additional medication. I wrote an order for the nurse to give him a placebo injection of 1 cc. of saltwater. The nurse told me that she could not follow that order because, by the order of the clinical director, we were not allowed to use placebo medications. This was strange, because as an intern in general medicine we had used placebos when we thought that the patient was feigning pain.

I asked the clinical director, who was my mentor, for the reason prohibiting the use of placebos. He said, "Abe, long before man developed the ability to speak, we communicated the way animals do, by scents, body language, and a variety of other non-verbal methods.

"When we developed verbal communication, that was superimposed upon the older non-verbal forms, but it did not eliminate them. Even now, we communicate non-verbally. It is just that our verbal communication obscures the non-verbal.

"You have conscious control of what you say, but you do not have voluntary control over non-verbal communication. If you give the patient a placebo, your verbal communication is, 'I am giving you something,' but your non-verbal communication is, 'I am giving you nothing.' You are sending your patient contradictory messages, which diminishes his trust in you and undermines the doctor-patient relationship, which is the only tool we have in psychotherapy."

I believed my mentor was right, and concluded that I cannot lie, not because it is ethically wrong, but rather because I cannot be a good liar. My involuntary non-verbal communication will betray the truth. Ever since then, I have avoided "white lies." These are easy to justify, but they can subvert any meaningful relationship.

There are times that I have made mistakes in therapy. Instead of covering them up, I admitted them. I have never sacrificed a patient's trust in me.

Some people think that they can get away by lying. It may work for the short term, but the long term effects are detrimental to any relationship.

THE THERAPIST'S CONVICTIONS

A therapist cannot expect a patient to accept anything that the therapist himself is unsure of. During World War II, a family in my father's congregation received word that their son, who was in the European theater of war, was missing in action. The family was devastated, assuming that he had been killed. My father tried to keep up the family's hopes, telling them that he may be a prisoner-of-war and that he would return when the war was over.

Every week, my father would visit the family, supporting them and offering them hope. When the war was over, it was discovered that their son had indeed been a prisoner-of-war. When the son returned to his army base, he found a stack of letters waiting for him. These were letters from my father, written once a week.

Prior to visiting the family, my father wrote a letter to the son, to reinforce his own belief that the son was alive. Unless he believed this strongly, his reassurance to the family would have been ineffective. He had to convince himself before he could expect the family to be hopeful.

An analogous incident is reported about Mahatma Ghandi. There was a young boy who was diabetic, and the parents could not convince him to stop eating sweets, which endangered his life. Inasmuch as the boy had a hero worship for Ghandi, the parents felt that he would accept instruction from Ghandi.

Getting to Ghandi was time-consuming and expensive. When Ghandi heard their request, he told them to return in two weeks. The parents' pleas not to delay were futile.

Two weeks later they returned to Ghandi, who took the boy aside and told him gently but firmly that he was not to eat sweets. The parents asked Ghandi why he did not do this two weeks earlier. Ghandi said, "Because two weeks ago,

I was eating sweets myself. It was only after I abstained for two weeks that I could tell your son that he must abstain."

We cannot expect of others more than we expect of ourselves.

PSYCHOTHERAPY OF PSYCHOSIS

Whereas psychotherapy of a variety of emotional problems can be effective, it is much different with psychosis. In psychosis, the patient has essentially broken with reality, and any attempt at logical reasoning is apt to fail. For example, a psychotic person may have the delusion that every move of his is being photographed and recorded by an international organization, and that his house is bugged. He may feel that he is under surveillance by automobiles that circle his block. Trying to convince him that this is a delusion is usually futile. You may point out to him that there is no possible reason why anyone would want to do these things, but he will reject this. He is certain that his ideas are true.

The medications that are currently used to treat psychosis may mitigate some of the symptoms, but as yet, there is no medication that eliminates the psychosis.

There are some anecdotes of rather unusual treatment techniques that have been effective, and from these I have learned to try to tailor therapy to the particular patient.

The rabbi of Talna was known for his ability to help psychotics. One person was brought to him who functioned normally, except that he had the delusion that he was the Messiah, and there was no budging him from this. When they brought him to the rabbi of Talna, the latter asked him, "Do you know who I am?"

"Of course," the man said. "You are the rabbi of Talna."

"Do you know that I have prophetic powers?" the rabbi asked.

"Yes," the man said, "everyone knows that you are Divinely inspired."

"Then wouldn't I know the identity of the Messiah?" the rabbi asked.

The man answered, "You must know then that I am the Messiah."

"But I have never revealed this to anyone. Just as I have never revealed my secret, you, too, must guard your secret assiduously. Do not reveal it to anyone, and neither will I."

The man never again mentioned to anyone that he was the Messiah and was able to live a normal life.

I was challenged by the case of a man who suffered a psychotic break during the Korean War. Upon returning home, he was repeatedly hospitalized, receiving a variety of treatments including intensive psychotherapy for several years. The family felt that he was never going to recover, but before placing him in a long-term facility, they wanted one more evaluation.

I met the man within an hour of his admission. He said, "Why is everyone here so angry at me? I didn't do anything to anyone. I just came."

Later that day I entered his room, where his dinner tray was untouched.

"Aren't you hungry?" I asked.

The man answered, "I can't eat. I don't have a mouth."

"Of course you have a mouth," I said.

"I don't feel I have a mouth," the man said.

At that point, it occurred to me that I had to take an unusual course. I said to him, "Look, you have been under the care of some of the finest psychiatrists in the country for the past ten years. If they could not get the crazy ideas out of your head, I'm not even going to try.

"But I think you can be helped to live a normal life. Listen carefully.

"For most people," I said, "their thoughts and their feelings are congruent. They *know* they have a mouth and they *feel* they have a mouth. Your problem is that your thoughts and feelings go in two separate directions. You *know* you have a mouth, but you don't *feel* it. Your thoughts are o.k., but your feelings are sick.

"All the other psychiatrists tried to help you change your feelings, and that didn't work. I don't think I can change your feelings. But I'll tell you what you must do. Ignore the feelings, and operate according to the facts as you know them.

"You don't feel you have a mouth. I believe you. That is a sick feeling, so you must ignore it. But intellectually you *know* you have a mouth. I want you to pick up that food and put it where you *know* your mouth is."

The man did exactly that, and finished his tray.

Then I said, "When I first met you, you felt that everyone here was angry at you, but you knew it couldn't be so because you had just come and had not done anything to anyone. So, you *knew* that they could not be angry at you, yet you *felt* that they were. That's another example of your feelings not being in harmony with the facts.

"If you can manage to ignore your feelings and live according to the facts as you know them, you may be able to stay out of mental hospitals."

The man said, "Oh, so that's how it is!"

I said, "Exactly! That's how it is."

From then on there continued a therapy consisting of twenty or thirty minutes a day. Whenever he would express a psychotic idea, I would say, "Arnie, that's a crazy thought. Ignore it! Live according to the facts."

After two months of this strange therapy, Arnie was able to leave the hospital. He rented a nearby apartment and came in every day for a brief session. He gradually learned to ignore his feelings and function according to his cognition, or knowledge of the facts. He did not have to be re-hospitalized for the first time in ten years!

In the "Stories" section of this book, I present another therapeutic entrance into the world of the psychotic. It was from such anecdotes and stories that I was able to learn something about an approach to a psychotic patient.

ABSURD PROBLEMS MAY BE DISMISSED

I am indebted to a rabbinical colleague for this technique. If a problem that has its origin in reality is so exaggerated that it becomes absurd, a person may be able to dismiss it. I may worry about being able to pay my bills this month, and may even lose sleep over it. However, if I were told that I had somehow incurred a debt of sixty-five billion dollars, it would not cause me any sleepless nights. That amount is so far out of reality that it doesn't even bother me.

I applied this technique to a woman whose husband complained that she had become housebound and withdrawn. She had received radiation treatment for a lesion on her nose, which had resulted in a prominent blemish that would, with time, disappear. She refused to allow anyone to see her because of this disfigurement. Her husband told her that people would not think she was ugly because of this blemish, but she remained self-conscious and isolated herself. It took much cajoling to bring her to my office.

When she told me about the problem that she was literally defaced by this blemish, I said to her, "I knew all about the spot on your nose. It was the lead story this morning on the NBC, CBS, ABC and CNN newscasts. The commentators talked about nothing else other than the spot on Esther's nose. They showed pictures taken by the astronauts in the space shuttle. It was the topic of the day in the United States Congress. When I came to the office this morning, the parking lot attendant and the elevator operator asked me, 'Did you hear about the spot on Esther's nose?' Of course it makes you isolate yourself. After all, no one is talking about anything else."

Esther laughed. "Oh, come on," she said, "you and your silly stuff. That's crazy."

I said, "It's just as crazy as your thinking that anyone gives a damn about that spot on your nose. I'm sorry to offend your ego, Esther, but no one really cares about your nose."

The absurdity of my exaggeration accomplished what logic could not, and Esther stopped behaving as though her nose was the center of the universe.

This can be a useful technique when applied judiciously.

SELF-AWARENESS AND SELF-ESTEEM

SEEKING AN IDENTITY

Among my favorite folk tales are the stories of "the wise men of Chelm." These stories are about a group of villagers who were remarkably stupid in a quaint sort of way.

Psychology stresses the importance of having an identity. Psychotherapists often try to help people "find themselves." A popular psychological theme is "Who am I really?" This story of the wise men of Chelm lends a perspective to this issue.

One day, a citizen of Chelm was at the public bathhouse. It suddenly dawned upon him that without clothes, most people look alike. He became quite anxious with the thought, "When it comes time to go home, how will I know which one is me?"

After pondering this a bit, he came up with a brilliant solution. He found a piece of red string and tied it around his great toe. He was now distinctly identifiable.

Unfortunately, in the process of sudsing and showering, the red string fell off his foot, and when another bather stepped on it, it stuck to his foot.

When it was time to leave, the first bather looked at his foot, and seeing nothing on it, was perplexed. Then he noticed the other man with the string on his foot. He approached him and said, "I know who you are, but can you tell me, who am I?"

Some people seek an identity by having the equivalent of a red string. Their identity is the luxury automobile in the driveway or the impressive façade on their mansion. But this is hardly an internal identity. What happens if one sells the car? Does the identity go along with it?

It is not much different if one's identity is, "I am a doctor" or "I am a lawyer." That is a description of what one *does* rather than what one *is*. If one's only identity is "I am a doctor," then one shares an identity with myriads of other doctors, but one does not have an individual identity.

The Chelmite's folly taught me something about identity seeking. I also found that a person with a true identity has a good self-awareness, which is conducive to self-esteem. His ego is not threatened by accepting teaching from everyone, as the following story illustrates.

TO BE ALWAYS TEACHABLE

The Talmud was so right about learning from everyone. Here is another quote from this treasure trove. "I learned much from my teachers, more from my peers, and most from my students." Some people's pride does not allow them to take instruction from anyone other than an acknowledged master. That is a serious mistake. In the medical hierarchy, doctors are superior to nurses. I learned things from nurses that doctors could not teach me.

I recall a man who came to the emergency room complaining of severe tremors. His hands were visibly shaking. The nurse called me aside and told me to have him extend his right hand, but I should watch the left hand. I did so, and while his extended right hand was shaking, his left hand was perfectly still. This man was putting on an act to get sedative medication. None of my instructors had taught me this way of detecting a malingerer.

The pride that prevents a person from learning from people who may be less educated than himself is nothing but an ego phenomenon. A person who has an inflated ego is usually someone with low self-esteem, who defensively makes himself out to be superior than others. People who know they are competent have no problem accepting teaching from those beneath them. They are the wise whom the Talmud says learn from everyone.

I was in my fourth month of psychiatric training when I received a call from a relative in New York. Since I was in psychiatric training, the family assumed I was the expert. She said that her husband was severely depressed, and asked what she should do. I suggested she consult a psychiatrist in New York. At that time I was reading the text on physiologic treatment of depression, written by the foremost authority on the subject, Dr. Lothar Kalinowsky. I told my relative to try to get an appointment with Dr. Kalinowsky.

Several days later, my secretary told me I had a call from Dr. Kalinowsky.

He had examined my relative, and felt that his severe depression required electroshock treatment, and wanted my opinion. I said, "Dr. Kalinowsky, I am not a psychiatrist. I am just in my fourth month of training, and whatever I know about electroshock is from your text."

Dr. Kalinowsky retorted, "Yes, I know electroshock, but you know this patient better than I do."

I said, "I can only tell you this. He is a brilliant man with a severe inferiority complex. He has avoided taking positions of responsibility for fear that he might fail. Although electroshock may relieve his depression, he is likely to say, 'I cannot take on any position of responsibility. They have tampered with my brain.'"

Dr. Kalinowsky admitted, "Yes, you are right. We cannot use electroshock."

I hung up the phone and promptly went to the chief of the department of psychiatry. "Guess who called me for consultation," I said, and told him about the call.

The chief smiled and said, "Abe, the only doctor who would consult a first year resident is the person who wrote the book. He has no fear that asking the advice of a beginner would reflect negatively on him. Doctors who refuse to ask advice from subordinates are those who are insecure."

At an AA meeting in a rural area, the speaker said, "I couldn't find a sponsor. I am sober for twenty-seven years, and my sponsor who was sober longer than me died. I couldn't find anyone around here who was sober longer than me to be my sponsor.

"Then someone said to me, 'Why does your sponsor have to be sober longer than you? All you need is someone with good sobriety who can be objective and recognize when your thinking is wrong.'

"I realized this guy was right. My insistence on taking guidance only from someone sober longer than me was an ego trip. I now have a sponsor who's been sober for ten years, and that's o.k."

This rather uneducated man had better insight than some people with multiple degrees. If I can overcome false pride, I will be able to learn something from everyone.

TO BE FREE

I was attending a Caduceus meeting (a meeting of recovering physicians). This was the first meeting for a surgeon, who had been mandated by the hospital administrator to take action to stop drinking. He had come into the emergency room one night clearly under the influence of alcohol.

The surgeon was belligerent. This was mid-December. "There are parties all over the place. Everyone is having a good time. It's not fair that I should be completely deprived of drinking. I don't think I am an alcoholic," he said.

One of the other physicians, who was ten years sober, said, "That's not the way I look at it. I did not want to give up my right to drink. Because I often drank too much, I tried to devise various ways to control my drinking so that it did not become excessive. When each way failed, I tried another way. My constant battle to control my drinking exhausted me, and it actually took the pleasure out of drinking.

"When I found out I was an alcoholic, it was a feeling of relief. There was no point in my trying to find ways to control my drinking. I had a disease which made it impossible for me to control it. I wasn't responsible for having that disease, and I admit I was a bit angry at why I was different than other people. Then I realized that I treat a number of diabetics. It's not their fault that they are diabetics. They have to live with their disease, and if they accept it and follow my instructions, they can have happy lives. There is not much logic in being angry for being diabetic."

Some people are critical of AA for using terms such as "surrender" or "powerless." This doctor's comments clarify that these are not terms of character weakness any more than is a diabetic's inability to produce sufficient insulin.

One veteran in recovery said, "There are control centers for everything in the brain. My control center for milk is in good condition. I never have more than one glass of milk a day. My control center for alcohol is on the blink. Nothing I can do to repair it."

If we realize what our physiological limitations are, we will not exhaust ourselves in trying to do the impossible. This sets us free from seeking endless ways to do what is beyond our means. Understood in this sense, accepting powerlessness over alcohol or some other things can set us free.

People who are "control freaks" may not realize that they have lost their freedom. Why? Because it is factually impossible to control other people. We may *think* we can control other people, but this is an illusion.

When you turn the steering wheel of your automobile, you are controlling which way it goes. If you are riding a horse and you wish to turn, you pull on the rein and the horse turns in the desired direction. Have you controlled the horse? Not really. Your pulling on the rein caused the horse discomfort as it pulled the bit in its mouth. To avoid the pain, the horse turned. Essentially, you made the horse an offer that was hard to refuse. However, if the horse was very hungry and saw a pile of hay in the other direction, it is possible that it might have ignored your command.

We may think that we control our children, our spouses or our employees. The fact is that we do not really control them. We just make them an offer that is hard for them to refuse. If circumstances change so that it is easier for them to refuse the offer, they may indeed do so.

A "control freak" is not a free person. He functions under the illusion that he can control people and is driven to do so. If he could realize, like the doctor with the alcohol, that he is really powerless over other people and his control is limited to the circumstances which make it hard for others to refuse his offer, then he might find more constructive and more pleasant ways of relating to them.

To be free in this sense requires a healthy ego. A person with good self-esteem does not have to be in control of other people.

We value freedom highly. The doctor's comment that accepting powerlessness can set one free has been of great help to me.

FORGIVING OURSELVES

In recovery from alcoholism, the AA program requires one to make a list of all the people one had harmed and to make amends to them if possible. One recovering alcoholic painstakingly made a list of all the people he had harmed or offended during his drinking years. He showed the list to his sponsor who said, "This list is incomplete."

The man said, "How can you say it's incomplete? How would you know whom I had harmed?"

The sponsor said, "You didn't put yourself at the top of the list."

When this man related this to me, it struck me as being true. Whenever we do something wrong, we harm ourselves.

We need to make amends to ourselves. We can do this by realizing what had led us to do the wrong act, and then change ourselves so that we will not do that act again.

I attended an AA meeting at which the speaker was a man who was celebrating the twentieth anniversary of his sobriety. He began his talk by saying, "The man I once was, drank. And the man I once was will drink again.

"I wasn't born a drunk. My character and personality developed in a way that led me to drinking. I can stay sober only as long as I don't go back to being the person that I was before I started drinking. If I ever go back to being that person, I will drink again."

These remarks electrified me. Whenever we do something wrong, we may feel guilty and resolve never to repeat that act. But that is not enough. How is it that we were able to do that wrong act? What defect was there in our characters that made that act possible? We must do a thorough soul-searching to discover that defect and do whatever it takes to rid ourselves of it.

When we eliminate character defects, we change our personality. We are not the person we once were. This new person is incapable of doing that wrong act. This awareness should enable us to forgive ourselves for that act. The new person that we have become should not be held *morally* responsible for what that old person did.

Of course, if that "old person" had injured someone, the "new person" must nevertheless make compensation for what the "old person" did. The character transformation does not cancel the debt. But if we have made the necessary amends and changed our character so that we would not repeat the wrong act, we should be able to forgive ourselves.

FROM LITERATURE

EVEN GREAT MINDS ARE NOT INFINITE

Our generation has been swamped with information in amounts that previous generations could not even dream of. With the touch of a finger, the internet can deliver more information than can fit into the Library of Congress. Internet addicts have an inexhaustible amount of data available to them. While the benefits of this are evident, there is also a down side: *information overload.*

One of the psychological theories about schizophrenia is that it is due to an "input overload." At any one moment, we are bombarded by many, many stimuli, most of which we ignore. For example, you are focusing on what you are reading, but you are not aware of the weight of the book on your hands unless you direct your attention to it. If you think about your shoes, you can feel that they are on your feet. If you listen for the sound of traffic outside your window, you will hear it. All these stimuli and many more impact on your sensory system at every moment. However, because you are focused on what you are reading, you ignore the sensations of the weight of the book, your shoes on your feet and the sounds of the traffic.

What would happen if you could not be focused? You would be aware of a million different stimuli at every moment, and that massive overload would so confuse you that you would not be able to think of any one thing. Fortunately, the mind has a "filtering system," which blocks awareness of all extraneous stimuli and allows you to focus. The theory is that in schizophrenia the filtering system is not functioning, and the person cannot possibly think clearly because his mind is overwhelmed.

Even the normal mind with an intact filtering system is subject to overload. If we try to know too much, we may become unknowledgeable about anything.

I was first introduced to this important concept by Sherlock Holmes. Yes, the famous detective. Dr. Watson expressed his amazement that Holmes was unaware of the Copernican theory that the earth revolves around the sun rather than the reverse. Every child beyond third grade knows this.

Holmes said, "No, I am not aware of it. Now that you have told me about it, I shall do my utmost to forget it."

"Forget it?" Watson exclaimed, "Why would you want to forget it?"

"My dear Watson," Holmes said, "my concept of the mind is that it is like a large cabinet with many drawers into which you can put whatever material you choose. Once all the drawers are filled, you cannot put anything more in until you first remove something from a drawer and make room for it. Therefore, a person should fill the drawers with only that material that is of use to him. Filling the drawers with irrelevant material will not allow him to store useful information.

"For what I do, it is totally irrelevant whether the earth revolves around the sun or the sun revolves around the moon. I must avoid cluttering my mind with useless information so that I can retain information that is important to me."

I may not agree with the model of the mind being a cabinet with drawers, but I believe that the principle is valid. If we absorb data that are irrelevant, we may not be able to focus adequately on what is important to us.

Whether at the keyboard of the computer or browsing in a bookstore, I must limit my intake to what is most relevant to me. Otherwise, I may become a victim of information overload.

"DOCTOR" CHARLES SCHULZ

Doctor Charles Schulz? You mean the cartoonist who created Snoopy and Charlie Brown? What kind of a doctor was he?

Charles Schulz, or as he was known to his friends, Sparky, was never trained to be a doctor of anything, but his grasp of human nature surpassed that of many highly educated psychiatrists and psychologists. He had the uncanny ability to illustrate some difficult concepts in a few frames of a cartoon strip.

I sometimes lecture about the frenetic pace of life we have adopted in the United States. We are always in a hurry, even when it makes no sense. I regularly see drivers cutting in front of me in traffic, taking some dangerous risks. At the next stop light, my front bumper is just inches away from the reckless driver's back bumper. He gained nothing by his impatience. But even if one does gain a few blocks and gets to his destination twenty-five seconds earlier, is it worth the risk? But we don't think like that. We are obsessed with speed. Our marvelous technology, with jet planes, fax machines, e-mail, instant foods and microwave ovens has eroded any tolerance of delay.

Sparky has a cartoon strip where Sally wakes up Charlie Brown. "Wake up, big brother," she says.

Charlie Brown sits up. "Wake up? What for?"

"So you can get an early start," Sally says.

"But I'm not going anywhere," Charlie Brown says.

"That's a shame," Sally says. "You could have been the first one there."

Schulz has encapsulated our frenetic culture in this single strip. Faster is better. Why? Because. Getting somewhere fast is more important than where you're going.

I have asked several business people, if a new copying machine were to come out that could make two hundred copies a minute instead of sixty, would they buy it? Invariably they say yes, they want to keep up with the state of the art.

"And when did you ever really need more than twenty copies a minute?" I ask. They admit that they never have, but that doesn't stop them from spending thousands of dollars for a machine that can do it faster.

Sparky's cartoon teaches us how unreasonable we can be.

During my psychiatric training, we did not learn anything about "behavior modification." This is a system of therapy based on the theory (it's really more than a theory) that behavior that is rewarded will be repeated, and behavior that is punished will be discontinued.

Charles Schultz has two characters: Marcie, who is very studious, and Peppermint Patty, who never gets a grade above D minus. Marcie complains to Charlie Brown that because Peppermint Patty felt so bad about failing, her father tried to cheer her up by taking her on a trip to Europe. "I got straight A's on my report card," Marcie says. "You know where I'm going? Nowhere." Schulz cleverly illustrates the folly of rewarding failure rather than success.

Much later, when I began working with addicts, I learned this principle. Addicts often get into trouble with the law, and well-intending family members bail them out. How can you expect one to overcome the addiction when you reward it?

Recently, Sparky's cartoon strips that antedated "Peanuts" were published. Among them was a cartoon that encapsulated the theory of Cognitive Therapy.

For decades, psychotherapy was based on Sigmund Freud's psychoanalytic theory. Essentially, if a patient could be helped to understand the origin of his symptoms, he would be relieved of them. This therapy necessitated a long, arduous search into the patient's remote past, trying to discover the ideas hidden in the subconscious mind which were causing the symptoms.

More recently, "cognitive psychology" has come to the fore. This school holds that a person's problems are due to his faulty perception of reality. Therapy is directed at correcting these distorted perceptions.

A picture is worth a thousand words. This cartoon says it all.

FROM PULPIT...TO COUCH

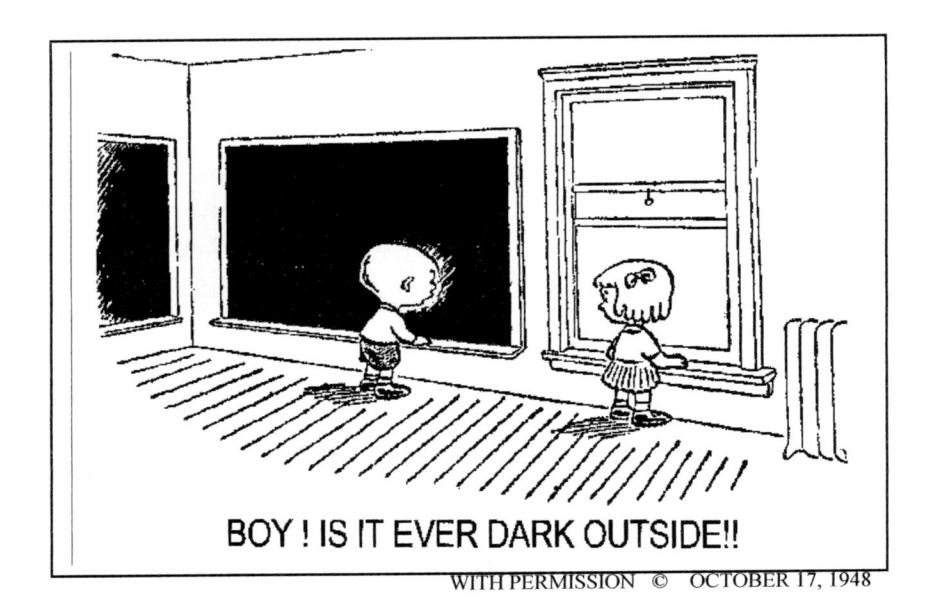

BOY! IS IT EVER DARK OUTSIDE!!

WITH PERMISSION © OCTOBER 17, 1948

If you have the mistaken idea that a blackboard is a window, the world will look awfully dark.

THE DISCOMFORT ZONE

Several years after I had completed my psychiatric training, I came across an article written by Dr. Frieda Fromm-Reichman, which had not been published during her lifetime. Dr. Fromm-Reichman noted that whereas the psychiatric literature frequently discussed anxiety, depression, and any number of symptoms, she was unable to find a single article on "loneliness." She concluded that loneliness is so distressing a feeling that even psychiatrists and psychologists feel threatened by it. It may arouse their own feelings of loneliness, which they would rather avoid. As I reflected on my psychiatric training, I realized that loneliness had never come up for discussion.

Realizing the validity of Dr. Fromm-Reichman's observation, I made it my business to ask my patients, "Do you ever feel lonely?" This inquiry has produced valuable information about the patient's emotional condition, and patients have helped me understand much about loneliness.

There is a difference between being "alone" and being "lonely." You may be amidst fifty thousand people in a sports stadium. You are certainly not alone, but you may be very lonely. None of those fifty thousand people care about you. When no one cares about you, you feel lonely. When a child falls and scrapes his knees, mother washes off the dirt and kisses the wound. That does not diminish the pain, but does take away the loneliness. What loneliness? The loneliness of thinking, "No one cares about my pain."

When I joined my father's congregation as assistant rabbi, I alternated with my father visiting hospitalized patients. I visited a patient who was several days post-operation. He said to me, "Nothing the doctors were giving me took away the pain, but when your father came in, it was like magic. The pain was gone." My father was a very caring person.

Pharmacologists say that morphine works differently from anesthetics. Anesthetics actually block the pain sensation. Morphine does not eliminate the pain sensation, but the patient does not feel the sensation as distress. Careful questioning of the patient may elicit the comment, "I still feel what I felt, but it doesn't bother me." Pain is a physical sensation, but the distress of pain is a psychological phenomenon. Loneliness may cause the pain to produce much distress. By eliminating the loneliness, sincere caring may diminish the distress sensation of pain.

Certainly in psychological problems, loneliness is a major factor. In psychiatric training we were cautioned about caring too much for the patient, because if we were to feel too much for him, we might lose the objectivity necessary for effective treatment. I'm not sure this is always correct. While a psychotherapist should guard against becoming over-involved with a patient's problem, he should nevertheless not deprive the patient of the caring that can diminish his loneliness.

FROM PEERS AND FRIENDS

DON'T TREAT HEALTH

It can be very frustrating for a psychiatrist who sees a patient weekly for two years and yet feels that he has made no progress. And the patient is as unhappy as ever. The logical thing to do is to take the case to a colleague who can provide a fresh look. "Here is the patient's history and all the pertinent data. Here's what I've done in therapy. There's been no progress in two years. What am I doing wrong?"

That is exactly what I did with this patient, who said, "Doctor, I understand everything perfectly. I know why I got to feel this way because of the things that happened in my growing years. Everything makes perfect sense. The problem is, I don't feel any different."

My colleague listened attentively, then said, "Abe, let me tell you a little story.

"You remember 'The Great Houdini,' who boasted that there did not exist a lock that he could not open. They once put Houdini in a box wrapped in iron chains with multiple padlocks and threw him under the surface of an ice-covered river. A few minutes later, Houdini emerged on shore.

"One prison warden challenged Houdini that he had a cell from which he could not escape. Houdini accepted the challenge. The warden took him to the cell and closed the door. 'I'll be in your office in five minutes or less,' he said.

"Houdini used to swallow tiny instruments and regurgitate them. He began working on the lock of the cell door, expecting to open it in fifteen seconds. When he had failed to open it in forty-five seconds, he became concerned. He thought a bit, then attacked the lock anew, but was unsuccessful. Disappointed and tired, he leaned against the cell door, and it swung open! The reason he could not open the lock was because it had never been locked. The warden had played a trick on him. Even Houdini could not unlock a lock that wasn't locked in the first place.

"Abe," my colleague said, "we are doctors and we treat disease. We cannot cure a person if he's not sick. I suspect that there is no particular pathology responsible for your patient's unhappiness. He is just discontented with the world the way it is. Disliking reality is an attitude, not a sickness. We can't treat it."

They forgot to teach me this in my psychiatric training. They taught me that all unhappiness was pathological and amenable to psychiatric treatment. If the unhappiness was not treatable with medication, then we had to delve into the patient's history, especially his childhood, to find what caused him to be this way. This is indeed true in some cases, but not in all cases.

People who have negative attitudes may just have to be apprised of reality. This can be better done by a competent counselor, perhaps a pastoral counselor who does not focus on pathology.

My colleague taught me a valuable lesson. *If the person you are treating is not getting better, take another look. He might not be sick.*

SMILING IS GOOD FOR YOU

We are often urged to greet people with a smile. "Keep smiling" is common advice. It makes contact with people more pleasant. It is generally assumed that when you smile, it elevates your mood a bit.

At a psychiatric convention, I was sitting across the table from a psychiatrist who periodically raised the corners of his mouth with his hand. I thought this was some kind of compulsive ritual. Even psychiatrists are not immune from obsessive-compulsive disorders.

The psychiatrist must have guessed my curiosity and he explained, "It has been proven that when you smile, it is the particular contraction of the facial muscles that causes the mood elevation. Today, I don't have anything to smile about, so, to lift my mood, I manufacture a smile by raising the corners of my mouth. Try it. It works!"

That came to me as a revelation. I now smile even when I don't feel like smiling.

Smiling may be nature's antidepressant.

WHEN SELFISHNESS IS GOOD

Parents frequently make sacrifices for their children and that's o.k. However, parents may sometimes sacrifice *themselves* for their children, and that can be counter-productive.

My father was a fanatic parent. If he saw me shoveling snow, he would take the shovel from me and do the shoveling. There was no arguing with him that it was perfectly safe for me to shovel snow, whereas for him it was a strain on his heart. He could not see that it was much more to my advantage to have a father than to be spared the work of shoveling snow.

It is not unusual for me to meet with parents who are making the same mistake. I learned something from a flight attendant that has been very helpful.

Most people have been on an airplane. I remind them of the flight attendant's instructions: "If the pressure in the cabin drops, oxygen masks will drop from the compartment above your seat. Place the mask over your nose and mouth and breathe normally. *If you are travelling with a child, put your own mask on first and then assist the child.*" The reason for this is that if you attend to the child first while you are deprived of oxygen, you may put the mask over his ear rather than over his nose and mouth, and you will actually be harming the child by your devotion to him.

We should realize that if we are in a position to be of help to someone, we must take proper care of ourselves first, because if we are rendered helpless, we cannot be of help to anyone else.

Isn't taking care of yourself first being selfish? Yes, but this is a good kind of selfishness.

A WISE GUIDELINE

Sometimes people may say something that is much more meaningful than they had intended. One such incident happened when I visited Vancouver.

One of the tourist attractions in Vancouver is a rope bridge which spans over a deep chasm. The narrow bridge is not fixed or anchored and it sways with the wind. Some brave souls were traversing the bridge, but as I looked down at the chasm below which appeared to be thousands of miles deep, my feet froze. I was paralyzed with fear. I was in a dilemma. My wife was crossing the bridge fearlessly, and I did not want to appear "chicken." Yet my fear was overwhelming.

A gentleman who was with us said, "Hold on to the rope railings and look upward toward the sky. Don't look down and you won't be frightened." I did as he said and succeeded in crossing the bridge.

The words he used remained with me, and I have applied them to numerous situations that were frightening. Don't focus on the object of your fear. Rather, look skyward, which I interpret as "Look up toward God."

This is not easy to do. Although I avoided looking down, I knew that the abyss beneath me was perilously deep. Just looking away from it would not do the trick. I had to look upward toward the sky.

Whenever I am confronted by a challenge that is fearsome, I think of these words. Look upward toward God. A strong faith in God can help one overcome even strong fears.

AGING HAS ITS ADVANTAGES

Here is something I learned from a sports announcer. We are very much a youth-oriented culture. A fifty-year old person who loses his job may find it difficult to get another job. Many companies prefer to hire younger people who are more energetic and less likely to have health problems that will require sick leave. Younger people are also likely to be more familiar with computer technology upon which so much of commerce depends. The value of experience may be overlooked.

I was listening to a radio broadcast of a Milwaukee Braves baseball game. The right fielder, Andy Pafko, was forty-four, which is the equivalent of a senior citizen in baseball. Indeed, this was the last season he played.

The batter hit a ball which was headed to be a sure home-run. Pafko, with his back against the right field wall, leaped up and snatched the ball just as it was about to clear the fence. The fans went crazy, and the announcer was screaming at the top of his voice, extolling the miraculous catch. "And think of it," he said, "Andy Pafko is forty-four! Can you imagine someone his age being able to jump that high?"

The co-announcer said, "You're making a mistake. Maybe a younger player could jump higher, but only someone with Pafko's experience could know exactly when to make the jump. A less experienced player would have missed the ball."

He was right. Youth certainly has its advantages, but so does experience. I have seen cases where younger physicians, equipped with state-of-the-art diagnostic equipment missed the correct diagnosis, while a septuagenarian physician who knew little about the highly sophisticated apparatus made the correct diagnosis primarily by listening carefully to the patient's history.

I am consulted by older people who feel that the rapid progress of modern technology has left them behind. I tell them about the unbelievable catch that Andy Pafko made in the late twilight of his career.

Of course, I have a personal interest in this. I am now beyond seventy. I identify with Andy Pafko. New medications and diagnostic tests are appearing faster than I can possibly absorb them, but I feel I have an expertise that more than compensates for the latest advances.

Some of that expertise came as a result of making mistakes, but learning from these mistakes has made me a better clinician.

A surgeon ran into some complications during an operation, and told his assistant to see if there were anyone in the surgical suite who could help him out. The assistant reported that the chief of surgery was there. "Should I call him?" he asked.

The surgeon said, "Hell, no. He wouldn't know what to do. He's never been in a mess like this before."

If you haven't made mistakes, your value is limited. Perfect people may not know how to help someone in trouble.

So I try to learn from everyone. Even from myself.

DON'T JUMP TO CONCLUSIONS

Some psychiatric patients suffer from paranoid psychosis. Psychotherapy is not of much help with them. No amount of reasoning can shake their conviction that they are the victims of a conspiracy to persecute them. However, some patients are not that far gone. They may indeed feel that others are doing things to them, but they may be amenable to logic.

With the latter patients I share an incident that happened to me. I was co-officiating at the funeral of a man who was a member in my congregation and also in another congregation. His funeral was held in the congregation of the other rabbi because it was larger and could accommodate more people.

I knew that the rabbi of the other congregation was not exactly enamored of me. We had appeared together on a panel, and the wit and style of my presentation had upstaged him. He was a good bit older than I, and it was evident that he resented this young upstart.

At the funeral, the host rabbi was first to deliver the eulogy. A few minutes into his address, the public address system failed, and no one beyond the first two rows could hear him. By the time it was my turn to deliver the eulogy, the problem had been corrected, and everyone could hear me.

What if it had been the reverse? What if the public address system had shut down when I was speaking? I would have been absolutely certain that the other rabbi had arranged it so that my speech should not be heard. What could have been more logical than that he did not wish to be upstaged again by me? No one could have convinced me that this was an accident.

Obviously, it was an accident, and so are many things that some people may interpret as hostile actions toward them. This experience has enabled me to make patients rethink their belief that they were being maligned.

Another incident of a somewhat similar nature happened when I celebrated my son's Bar Mitzvah. I said to a friend, "You didn't return your R.S.V.P. card. Aren't you coming?" My friend said, "I would have returned the card if I'd received an invitation."

I was stunned. I distinctly remember writing his address. I then discovered that another friend had not received an invitation. Both friends' names began with "R." I then checked my invitation list and called everyone whose last name began with "R." None of them had received an invitation. Obviously the group of invitations addressed to "R" people had been mislaid or had gotten lost in the mail.

Ever since then, if I don't receive an invitation to a friend's celebration, I go anyway. It is a mistake to conclude that they intentionally did not invite me.

We should be very cautious about jumping to conclusions. Even what may seem obvious may have another explanation.

A HELPFUL HINT

This doesn't have anything to do with psychiatric practice, but I just wish to pass along a piece of advice I received from a friend, for which I am most grateful.

I remember my father being kept up to all hours of the night by people who were pests. They talked and talked, never saying anything of substance. My father was too gentle a person to terminate the session.

I was given excellent advice. If someone hangs on to you and won't go away, ask him to lend you some money. In all likelihood, he won't come around as often. Or, if he is a person of meager means, lend him some money. In order to avoid your asking him to repay the loan, he will stay away.

Try it. It works.

INSANE OR NORMAL?

In my psychiatric training I was told that people who are delusional are insane, and people who are in touch with reality are normal. That should be obvious, but a recent recall of a childhood memory gives me second thoughts.

When I was five or six years old, Mr. Wobek attended my father's synagogue occasionally. He would come and leave before the worshippers came. Wobek wore a ten gallon hat and sported a carved cane. On one hand he wore a huge diamond ring, and on the other hand a large blue sapphire ring. He wore a stiffly starched shirt, and the buttons were green sapphire studs. He was a pleasant man. I would sit on his lap, and he would tell me stories about palaces, princes and presidents.

Wobek had at one time been very wealthy, and the precious gems he had sported then were genuine. He lost everything in the crash of 1929 and went insane, whereupon his wife left him. He withdrew from people, and had grandiose delusions that he was still a millionaire. (A millionaire of the 20's would be a billionaire today.) The huge rings and the sapphire studs were glass, but to a six year old child, there is no difference between diamonds and glass.

I listened, wide-eyed, to his stories. They were not totally untrue, because in his better days, he did associate with important people. Shortly before worshippers would arrive, he would tell me that he had to go, and that his driver would pick him up in a limousine. I was curious to see the limousine, and I watched Wobek walk *down to the bus stop*, where he indeed alighted into a very large and expensive vehicle that indeed had a driver.

A while back, I attended a gala social event. One wealthy lady was bedecked with diamond necklace, earrings, and rings. I made a comment that with all that jewelry she should be protected by a bodyguard. I was told that all the diamonds she wore were simulated. Her genuine diamonds are in a vault, and she never wears them.

Wobek and this lady both wore simulated gems. She was normal, whereas Wobek's doing so was crazy.

I have some difficulty figuring this one out. What is the purpose of having diamonds if you never take them out of the vault? Is that normal or insane?

... AND FROM PATIENTS

DEATH IS ALWAYS SUDDEN

I was on the staff of a state mental hospital, and a woman was admitted to my service who had been hospitalized previously. Before seeing her, I reviewed the chart of her earlier admission. Her husband had died of kidney failure, and for a long time had been a terminally ill patient in the Veterans Administration Hospital.

When I interviewed this woman, she related several things that she felt had brought on her depression. She said that her husband's sudden death had been a severe shock.

I said, "I'm sorry, but from what I saw in your record, your husband had been suffering from a terminal illness for a long time."

The woman said, "Oh, yes, that's true. But whenever death happens, it's still sudden."

This woman knew something that I, as a psychiatrist, did not know. I assumed that when someone is expected to die from a terminal illness, it is not sudden nor is it a shock. This woman set me straight. She was right. Regardless of how sick a person may have been, and even if death comes as a welcome relief from his suffering, it is always a sudden occurrence and may be a shock even if it is expected.

Our conscious mind operates according to logic. When something is expected for a long time, it is not sudden nor shocking. However, our emotions are mostly subject to our subconscious mind, which does not abide by logic. Shock is an emotional reaction, and to the subconscious, death is always sudden.

This is important in understanding a person's reaction to the death of a loved one. We may not think of it as a traumatic incident, hardly likely to result in a Post Traumatic Stress Disorder. This woman knew better. She did suffer from a Post Traumatic Stress Disorder as a result of her husband's "sudden" death.

When someone loses a loved one who had lingered with a terminal illness, we may think that they will not grieve excessively and will not need consolation and support. This is a mistake. They need closeness and consideration just as much as if the death had actually been sudden.

LOVE AND LIKE ARE NOT SYNONYMOUS

A sixteen-year-old young woman was admitted to my service in the psychiatric hospital. She said that if she is crazy, it is because her mother drove her crazy. Her mother was an unreasonable person who had never shown her any love and who was frankly abusive. She did not think that she could return home after leaving the hospital. Her father was very passive and never intervened to stop her mother's abusiveness.

After two weeks in the hospital, she requested a week-end pass. "What for?" I asked. "I want to see my mother," she said.

"I thought you wanted to get away from your mother," I said.

"I do. I can't live with her," she said.

"Then why do you want to go home to her?" I asked.

"Because I love her."

"From what you've been telling me, I didn't think that you loved her," I said.

"Of course I love her," the young woman said. "She is my mother, so I love her. I don't *like* her, because there is nothing about that woman that anyone can like."

My instructors had failed to tell me that there is a vast difference between liking someone and loving someone. Love is a more biological emotion, whereas "like" is much more of an intellectual feeling. I'm grateful to this young woman for having enlightened me.

We may think that "love" is an intensification of "like." We may say, "That's a nice outfit. I like it very much." We may also say, "I just *love* that dress," which means that one *likes* it much more than the outfit. But "like" and "love" are not merely different quantitatively. They are qualitatively distinct.

It is perfectly possible to love a person even if you don't like him at all.

TO BE ALWAYS CONSIDERATE

In my first year of psychiatric training, I worked on a closed, in-patient unit. One day, I was walking down the corridor, jingling the keys in my pocket, when one patient remarked, "I know you have the keys to this place. You can leave it and I can't. You don't have to rub it in."

I was not aware that my jingling of the keys could be taken as flaunting my authority and demeaning the patient. Heaven knows, that is the last thing I would have wanted to do. Yet, I inadvertently had hurt someone.

Is it possible that in my subconscious I really did want to flaunt my authority and that the patient was right? I have no way of knowing what lies in my subconscious. In any case, I am responsible for my behavior.

There is a folk saying, "If someone had a relative who was hung, do not say to him, 'You may hang your coat in the closet.'" Just the association of the word "hang" may be enough to evoke a painful feeling.

Recently, I received a joke via the internet. A man who was attending a convention registered at the desk, and the clerk gave him a name tag which read "Hello, my name is..." and asked him for his name so that she could fill it in on the tag. The man said, "Mary Jo Smith." The clerk said, "I mean what is *your* name?" Again the man said, "Mary Jo Smith." The clerk said, "I don't understand." The man said, "I went bankrupt. Everything is now in my wife's name."

I thought it was funny, and I passed it on. We were having dinner with some friends, and I was about to relate this joke to them, when I remembered that this man had indeed declared bankruptcy. To him the joke would have been painful rather than funny.

We should keep our wits about us. We feel bad if we accidentally spill hot soup on someone's clothes. We should be just as careful not to accidentally hurt someone's feelings.

THE BEAUTY OF LIGHT

This woman was not my patient. She was a ninety-six-year-old resident of a nursing home, who had not spoken a single word for over a year. No amount of cajoling could get her to speak. It was assumed she was suffering from senile dementia.

One of the candy striper volunteers, a young woman of fourteen, was assigned to sit with this woman. The old woman looked out the window, totally ignoring the young woman to engage her in conversation or in an activity. Nothing could distract her from looking out the window.

After an hour, the young woman had just about had it. She arose to leave, but couldn't help asking, "What are you looking at?"

The "demented" old lady looked at her and smiled, "Why, at the light, my child."

We, whose mental faculties are intact, probably never look at the light. It is with the help of the light that we can see things, and we focus our attention on the many things we see, but not on the light itself.

Isn't that strange? In the story of creation, the Bible says, "And God said, 'Let there be light,' and there was light. And God saw the light *that it was good.*" Stop and think for a moment. According to the account of creation, the light was the first thing created. There were no trees, no grass, no animals, no birds. *There was nothing to see but the light*, yet God saw that the light was good. There must be something intrinsically good about light, even if it has no practical application.

I never thought about this until I heard about the old woman's remark. Perhaps her mental condition was such that she could not focus on anything. All she saw was the light, and she felt that it was worth looking at.

We often think of wisdom as a kind of light. We speak of wise people as being "enlightened," and we may say that a person had a "bright" idea.

I think that many people do not value wisdom unless it has some practical application. Knowledge is of value only if it is useful. But the determination of what is morally right or wrong, good or evil, requires wisdom. True, the conclusions may not necessarily have a practical application. Perhaps this has contributed to an abdication of thinking about moral and ethical issues.

Maybe there is something we can learn from a ninety-six-year-old "demented" woman.

DIAMONDS

Sometimes people ask, "What made you choose to work with addicts?" In "My Teacher, Isabel," I related how I got *started* in this field. The following story is an example of why I *stayed* in it.

A number of years ago, I began a small rehabilitation program in Israel for ex-convicts who had been imprisoned for drug-related crimes. In a session with the first group of clients, I pointed out that there is a natural resistance to avoid damaging an object of beauty. Inasmuch as everyone knows that drugs are damaging, there should have been greater resistance to their taking drugs. The reason they did not have this resistance was because they had never considered themselves to be worthy and beautiful. I said that long-term recovery depends on developing self-esteem, so that one would not want to damage one's self.

One of the ex-convicts said, "How can you expect me to have self-esteem. I'm 34 years old, and sixteen of those 34 years have been spent in prison. When I get out of prison, no one will give me a job. When the social worker tells my family that I will be released in ninety days, they are very unhappy. I am a burden and an embarrassment to them. They wish I would stay in jail forever or even die. How am I supposed to get self-esteem?"

I said to him, "Avi, have you ever seen a display of diamonds in a jewelry store window? Those diamonds are scintillatingly beautiful and worth hundreds of thousands of dollars. Do you know what they looked like when they were brought out of the diamond mine? They looked like ugly, dirty pieces of glass, which anyone would think worthless.

"At the diamond mine, there is a *mayvin* [expert] who scrutinizes the ore. He may pick up a "dirty piece of glass" and marvel at the precious gem that lies within. He sends it to the processing plant, and it emerges as a magnificently beautiful, shining diamond.

"No one can put any beauty into a dirty piece of glass. The beauty of the diamond was always there, but it was concealed by layers of material that covered it. The processing plant removed these layers, to reveal the beauty of the diamond. They did not create the beauty, just exposed it.

"I may not be a *mayvin* on diamonds, Avi," I said, "but I am a *mayvin* on people. You have a beautiful soul within you, but it has been covered with layers of ugly behavior. We will help you get rid of those layers and reveal the beauty of your soul."

Avi stayed in the program for several months, then was in a transitional facility for eight months. After leaving, he found a job and remained free of drugs.

One day, Annette, the administrator of the program received a call from a family whose elderly mother had died, leaving an apartment full of furniture for which they had no use. They offered to donate the furniture to the rehabilitation program. Annette called Avi and said, "I have no way of getting that furniture here. Could you help us?" Avi assured her that he would get a truck and bring the furniture.

Two days later, Avi called Annette. "I am at the apartment," he said, "but there is no point in bringing the furniture. It is old and dilapidated."

Annette said, "I don't want to disappoint the family, Avi. Bring it here. Perhaps we can salvage some of it."

Avi loaded the truck and brought the furniture to the facility, which was on the second floor of a building. As he dragged an old sofa up the stairs, an envelope fell from the cushions. It contained 5000 shekels ($1800 US). This was money of whose existence no one knew, and the rule of "finders-keepers" could easily have been applied, especially by someone who used to break into a house for ten shekels.

Avi called Annette and told her about the money. "That's the family's money," she said. "Call them and tell them." The family graciously donated the money to the rehabilitation program.

On a subsequent visit to Israel, I met Avi at a function of the rehabilitation program, and that is when Annette told me the story about the 5000 shekels. I said to Avi, "Do you remember our first meeting when you did not know how you could ever have self-esteem? I told you that there was a soul, a beautiful diamond within you. Many people who never stole a penny would have simply pocketed the money. What you did was truly exceptional, and shows the beauty of the 'diamond' within you."

Several months later, Avi affixed a bronze plaque on the door of the rehabilitation center. It read *"**DIAMOND PROCESSING CENTER**."*

AFRAID OF PRAISE

No one likes to be put down, right? Everyone likes to be praised, right? Well, not always.

Celia was a drug-addicted nurse who had not been able to work for years. She requested treatment for her addiction because all her veins had collapsed from repeated heroin injections. For several months she had been injecting heroin into her muscles, and had developed dangerous abscesses. I had to send Celia to a hospital for a week to treat the infections.

Celia then entered the rehabilitation program, and after three weeks of not using drugs and eating nutritious meals, her appearance improved markedly. Meeting her in the lobby one day, I said, "Celia, you're really beginning to look good." She responded angrily with an obscene expletive.

The next day, Celia came to my office and apologized. "I'm sorry for what I said to you yesterday. You said something positive to me. I just didn't know how to handle that."

Celia's behavior over the years had elicited nothing but critical and insulting comments. She had become accustomed to these and knew how to respond. The first time she heard a word of praise, she was taken by surprise. She was totally unfamiliar with positive comments.

Celia taught me that people may prefer something with which they are familiar, regardless of how unpleasant it may be. This is why children who run away from an abusive parent often return home, knowing that they will be severely beaten. They are more comfortable with the familiar than with people whose behavior may be more pleasant, but is unpredictable.

People consult psychotherapists because of some type of distress. It is not at all unusual for them to refuse to make the changes that would improve their condition. Pain may actually be more pleasurable to them, and pleasure may be more painful.

BEWARE THE LABELING

I shall be forever indebted to two recovering drug-addicts who taught me something that I had not learned in my psychiatric training.

A young man was admitted to the psychiatric hospital in a catatonic state. He was mute, hardly moved and rarely blinked. He presented a picture of a classic catatonic schizophrenic.

Later that day I was visited by two recovering addicts. "We'd like to talk to you about B.J.," they said. "Please don't treat him like a schizophrenic."

"But he is schizophrenic," I said.

They said, "No, Doc. B.J. is crazy, but he is crazy like an addict is crazy. He'll be alright. Just don't give him any medicines. We'll take him to a Narcotics Anonymous meeting every day."

Although this sounded absurd to me, I agreed. Every day the two came and carried out this statue-like patient to a meeting, and brought him back several hours later. After two weeks, B.J. began talking, and a week later, he was perfectly normal, without any symptoms of schizophrenia.

Since then, I have had several patients who had been diagnosed as schizophrenic and treated for schizophrenia, who actually had a drug-induced psychosis, and whose treatment essentially consisted of keeping them off of drugs.

Unfortunately, diagnostic labels may stick to a person like the strongest adhesive cement. Once labeled "schizophrenic" or "bi-polar," the person may be treated as such *for the rest of his life*. Some psychiatrists may not elicit a history of drug use, or ignore it if they do. I teach psychiatric residents to carefully investigate the possibility of drug use and to withhold making any psychiatric diagnosis until the patient has been clean from all drugs and alcohol for at least four weeks.

What I learned from these two recovering addicts has saved several people's lives.

ACCEPTING HELP

It's quite easy to identify character defects in other people, but it's very difficult to identify them in yourself. A good rule of thumb is to try to look at yourself honestly when you see faults in others, and ask yourself, "Am I like that?"

One winter we had a spell of sub-zero weather. I was told that one of my patients, a woman who had been sober for about eight months had slept in an unheated apartment for several nights because her furnace had broken down. The repair people were overloaded and could not get to her furnace for several days. One of the women in AA said to her, "How silly! You could have stayed at my house for a few nights." She said, "Oh, no. I don't like to impose on anyone."

I called Grace and said to her, "You are doing so well in your recovery that I was hoping I would be able to ask you to work with a newcomer."

Grace said, "Please, Dr. Twerski, call on me at any time. I'll be glad to help."

I said "No, Grace, I guess I can't. If you are unable to accept help, you have no right to give it."

But then I had to look honestly at myself. I constantly try to help others, but in no way would I let anyone help me. Accepting help was a sign of weakness. I had to do everything myself, even when things were obviously too big for me to cope with alone.

This was in the days when I was struggling with my own self-esteem problem. As my self-esteem improved, I did not feel threatened by accepting help.

If you find yourself rejecting help, you may be where I once was. Low self-esteem is the result of an erroneous self-concept. Invariably, when you correct your distorted self-perception, your self-esteem improves and you can accept help gracefully.

MARRIAGE COUNSELING

You might think that marriage counseling would be a high priority in psychiatric training. After all, so many problems occur in marriage. Just look at the divorce rate in the U.S. Forty percent of marriages end up in divorce! Someone even quipped, "The leading cause of divorce is marriage." Strange, I received no instruction at all about marriage or spouse abuse.

I was left on my own to figure out how to handle marital strife. I could read some books on the subject. But one of the best insights came from a patient who told me that at one point, his marriage was in deep trouble.

"My wife and I had frequent spats," he said. "I never wanted to yield. It was a matter of pride. I was right even if I was wrong.

"Then one day it occurred to me that if I win an argument, that means that my wife lost it. But I didn't want to be married to a loser, so we stopped fighting."

Perhaps it was still a matter of pride that he did not want to be married to a loser, but it certainly is a much healthier result of pride than on insisting on being a winner.

DEPRESSED ABOUT?

Here's something I learned that was very important in my psychiatric practice. I learned it from a patient. That patient was *me*.

I received my psychiatric training in 1960, before much was known about the chemistry of emotions. The institute where I trained was wedded to Freudian psychology. We were taught that all depressions were due to a loss of some sort. The reasoning went like this: A loss results in being depressed. Therefore, every depression is due to a loss. But what if the depressed person had not sustained a loss? Never mind. He did suffer a loss, but was unaware of it. His *subconscious* was aware of the loss.

We were taught that the depression that frequently follows childbirth is because the woman has *lost* the pregnancy. But this is no loss. She very much wanted the child, and was so happy with it. Well, the reasoning went, her *conscious* mind was happy with the baby, but to her *subconscious,* delivering the baby was like losing a part of her body. I hate to admit that I bought into this theory.

In my second year of training, I became depressed. I couldn't think of what I might have lost. As the depression grew worse, I consulted one of my instructors. After listening to me, he said, "Abe, are you taking any medications?" I said, "Just something for hay fever, a decongestant." "Why don't you just stop the medication and let's see what happens." I stopped the medication, and within two weeks my depression disappeared. I later noted that one of the side effects of this medication could be depression.

I returned to my instructor. "What about the theory that depression is always due to a loss, either a conscious or subconscious loss?"

My instructor smiled. "There is no greater tragedy than a good theory being disproved by a fact."

Ever since then, psychiatry has advanced. It is now common knowledge that many depressions are the result of an imbalance in the body's chemistry. I found this out the hard way.

WHAT ELSE IS THERE?

As drug use among adolescents increased, there was a scramble for prevention programs. Sad to say, after several decades and billions of dollars spent on the "War on Drugs," we still cannot point to any prevention program that has really been effective.

I met with a number of adolescents, and one of them said, "They go around saying, 'Just say NO to drugs.' Why should I? What else is out there for me?"

This youngster enlightened me about the ineffectiveness of drug prevention programs. Drugs give a very pleasurable sensation. Kids don't see that there is anything that life can offer them that would give them real pleasure.

This young man set me to thinking, "What are we modeling for our children?" What is adult life about other than pursuit of pleasure? O.K., not everybody indulges in alcohol or drugs. But what motivates most people? They pursue pleasure in trying to make more money, get praise, enjoy good food, and, in brief, get as much fun out of life as possible.

Once I participated in a banquet tribute to a volunteer group. These were people who made it their business to cheer up "shut-ins." A "shut-in" is an elderly widow or widower who has not worked for a number of years, whose two children live hundreds of miles away, whose poor vision precludes driving a car and arthritis and emphysema curtail any physical activities. Shut-ins stay alone in their apartment, living in the misery of loneliness.

These volunteers would donate several hours a week to be with shut-ins, perhaps to drive them to the supermarket or a doctor's appointment, or take them for a pleasant drive or walk, or play a game with them. The theme of the banquet was "Doing Good Versus Feeling Good." It struck me that here we have the answer to the drug epidemic. If we would live our lives in a way that demonstrated that "feeling good" is secondary to "doing good," our youngsters might learn that there is something more important in life than pleasure.

Alas! The television is top-heavy with pursuit of pleasure. Very few commercials urge people to make "doing good" the primary focus of life.

The youngster who said, "What else is there?" put his finger on the problem.

THE NEED FOR AN IDENTITY

I've always felt that an identity and having self-esteem are important. Sometimes I'm asked, "With your busy schedule, how did you ever find the time to write forty-three books?" My answer is that I never wrote forty-three books. I've written one book, in forty-three different ways. Everything I wrote is an elaboration on the importance of self-esteem. Yet, I must admit that I did not grasp just how crucial having an identity is until I was taught this by. . . a prisoner.

There was a man in Pittsburgh who was an immigrant, arriving in the United States as a penniless young man of seventeen. He was a very shrewd businessman. He worked odd jobs, saved his money and bought a four-unit house. He continued to invest in real estate and eventually became very wealthy. He was charitable and active in community affairs. He had little formal education, and was essentially a self-made man.

This man had a son whom he sent to college. He was an average young man who lacked his father's entrepreneurial skills. He managed some of his father's properties, and although he did not lack for money, he was essentially a rent collector. Standing in his father's shadow, he felt completely effaced. He started a small business venture on his own which failed.

One morning the newspaper had the young man's picture on the front page. He had been arrested in a bank robbery. Bank robbery? For what? He had all the money he needed.

One of my jobs was doing psychiatric evaluations on prisoners. When they brought this young man in for an interview, he stretched out his hand and greeted me with a broad smile. "Hey, Doc, did you see my picture in the paper?"

That was it. He had finally achieved some recognition. He did not realize that he was not even a good criminal, bungling the attempted robbery. But so what? Now he had recognition.

This prisoner taught me just how desperate a person may become if he lacks an identity and self-esteem.

STORIES

BRIEF PSYCHOTHERAPY

There is much we can learn from stories.

In recent years, there has been a trend toward brief psychotherapy, a contrast to classical long-term therapy. This was not as much due to a change in psychiatric theory as to expedience. Insurance carriers simply refuse to cover more than a few sessions of therapy.

I came around to brief psychotherapy on my own. When I was in psychiatric training, I visited home, and my father was interested in what I was learning. When I told him that insight-oriented, psychodynamic psychotherapy may take several years, he was skeptical, and he told me the following story.

In Czarist Russia, the feudal system prevailed. Each nobleman had his fiefdom over which he had absolute rule. Most of these noblemen were ardent anti-Semites, and the Jewish population was subject to pogroms. If you've seen *Fiddler on the Roof,* you may have an idea of what a mild pogrom was like.

One nobleman, however, was a pacifist. He simply abhorred violence, and he did not allow any pogroms in his fiefdom. Some of the virulent anti-Semites in his fiefdom tried to provoke him to conduct a pogrom, but he consistently refused.

These trouble makers then fell upon an idea. This nobleman had a dog which was his constant companion. He loved that dog more than anything else in the world. They then said to him, "Your Lordship, you know that Jews are a very shrewd people. Why, they have a way of teaching a dog how to talk, but it is a well-kept secret. They would never reveal it to you, because you are not one of them. They will never admit this. They will give you all kinds of excuses, but the truth is that they would not reveal it to you because you are a gentile."

They had found the nobleman's Achilles' heel. He called in the leaders of the Jewish community and said, "You know how I have consistently protected you. My fiefdom is the only one in which there have not been any pogroms, and you have been able to live in peace and security.

"I have one favor to ask of you, and I know that in your gratitude you will not refuse me. My dog is my constant companion. We have a way of communicating with each other, but it is limited. If my dog could talk, it would give me the opportunity to converse with him, and that would be my Paradise. I know that you have a secret method of teaching a dog to talk, and I want you to grant me this one favor."

The Jewish community leaders were stymied. "Your Lordship, there is nothing in the world that we would not do for you. We owe our very lives to you, and if you would ask us to jump into a fire, we would not refuse you. However, what you are asking is impossible. There is no such thing as teaching a dog to talk."

The nobleman became irate. "So that is how you repay me for protecting you all these years from pogroms! You are a bunch of ingrates. I will hear none of your lies and excuses. You have thirty days to teach my dog how to talk, or every single Jew, from young to old, will be driven out of my fiefdom."

"But Your Lordship...," the Jewish leaders began to say.

The nobleman interrupted, shouting, "Silence! I will hear no more! Thirty days, or expulsion. Now leave here immediately."

The Jewish community was in agony. What can you do with a man who is seized by a delusion that a dog can be taught to talk? Any attempt to reason with the nobleman failed. He would not allow anyone into his palace unless they had come to teach the dog to talk.

The thirtieth day was nearing, and the Jews were loading all their belongings on wagons, ready to leave the fiefdom. On the thirtieth day, one of the lesser luminaries of the community, a humble shoemaker, said, "Let me talk with the nobleman."

The community leaders said, "Are you crazy? He is mad with this delusion. He will not listen to our learned rabbis. What can you say to him?"

The shoemaker said, "What do you have to lose? You are ready to leave, aren't you?" The leaders permitted him to try to reason with the nobleman, although it was certainly futile.

After an hour, the shoemaker emerged from the palace, with a dog on a leash. "Unpack the wagons, everybody! We're staying!"

"What do you mean 'we're staying'?" the community leaders said, "and what are you doing with that dog?"

The shoemaker said, "I told the nobleman that I would teach his dog to talk. I explained to His Lordship that a human child is much more intelligent than a dog. It takes about two or three years for a child to learn how to talk, so he must understand that it will take five or six years to teach a dog to talk."

"But what will happen at the end of six years?" the community leaders said.

"Relax!" the shoemaker said. "During the six years, *something* is bound to happen that will extricate us from this predicament. Within six years, perhaps I will die, or the dog will die or the nobleman will die. Within six years something will happen that will resolve this problem."

After my father finished the story, he said, "You are going to treat a patient for several years and then claim that your treatment helped him? Just think of how many things can happen in those years that may alter his life situation for the better.

"He may find a new job, he may marry, he may divorce, he may move away from meddling in-laws, his enemies may die, he may have children. Why, there is no limit to the kinds of things that may transpire during a period of several years. How can you take credit for his improvement?"

To me, this made good sense. I embraced brief psychotherapy a long while before the insurance companies mandated it.

ENTERING THE WORLD OF THE PSYCHOTIC

The following is a story by Rabbi Nachman of Bratslav. It has been cited frequently, and various interpretations have been given to the story. I see it as a therapeutic technique of entering into the world of the psychotic patient.

A young prince went insane. He had the delusion that he was a turkey. He sat nude under the table and ate whatever crumbs fell. The distraught king brought the finest doctors from the four corners of the earth, but no one could cure the prince of his delusion.

One day a wise man appeared, and told the king that he had a way of curing the prince. He took off his clothes and went under the table to where the prince was eating crumbs.

"What are you doing here?" the prince asked.

"What are you doing here?" the wise man asked.

"I'm a turkey," the prince said, "and I'm eating the crumbs that fall from the table."

"Well, I'm a turkey, too," the wise man said, helping himself to some crumbs.

Every day, the wise man sat naked under the table, eating crumbs and making small talk with the prince. Then one day, the wise man wore socks. "Why are you wearing socks?" the prince asked. "Turkeys don't wear socks."

"They sure do," the wise man said. "When their feet get cold, turkeys wear socks. Why should they suffer with cold feet?"

A few days later the wise man brought a pair of socks. "Here" he said to the prince, "you don't have to have cold feet."

Several days later, the wise man wore a shirt. "Why are you wearing a shirt?" the prince asked.

"Because I'm cold," the wise man said. "We turkeys are very smart. When we get cold, we put on a shirt."

Several days later, the prince put on a shirt that the wise man brought him. Eventually the prince was fully dressed.

One day, the wise man said, "I don't know why the people should have all the good food, and we turkeys must be satisfied with crumbs. I'm going to get some of the food from the table." Soon the prince was eating food from the table.

Very gradually, the wise man introduced item after item of normal living, until the prince's behavior was undistinguishable from that of any normal person. No one knew that in his heart, the prince thought he was a turkey.

I have no idea what point Rabbi Nachman was trying to make with this story. I can only tell you that it has helped me enormously in dealing with delusional people, whether it be the delusion of psychosis or the delusion of alcoholism.

CLOSED-MINDEDNESS

One of the greatest frustrations confronting the psychotherapist is being unable to overcome a patient's resistance to a valid interpretation or recommendation. People's behavior may be so ingrained that they have great difficulty in changing it.

One patient as she related her problem, said, "I'm so sorry for crying."

I responded, "There's nothing wrong with crying when you're hurting, and there's no need to apologize for doing so."

"I always apologize for everything," she retorted.

"It's time to stop that. If you haven't done anything wrong, don't apologize. O.K.?"

"Alright," she said. "I'll stop apologizing."

As she left the office, there was a man sitting in the waiting room. She said to him, "I'm sorry for taking so much of the doctor's time."

Sometimes you just can't win. I once mentioned this to my father, who, as a rabbi, was a natural, highly-gifted therapist. He told me the following story.

When the first locomotive was introduced in Europe, word about this amazing phenomenon came to a small village. When the villagers heard that there was a wagon that moves without horses attached to it, they howled with laughter. "How stupid can people be to believe that a wagon will move without horses!"

When the stories about the locomotive kept on coming, the villagers decided that they must debunk this myth by a personal investigation. They chose the most enlightened person in the village to go to the big city and see what makes people believe that a wagon can move without horses.

The representative returned and called a town meeting. "My friends," he said, "it is not a fantasy. It is true." He was greeted by a derisive booing. When this subsided, he said, "Let me explain."

He then drew on the board a diagram of the steam engine, showing how the fire turned the water to steam, which pushed up against a piston that was connected to wheels. Each time the steam pressure pushed against the piston, that caused the wheels to turn and the wagon to move.

A few of the villagers promptly understood, but many were bewildered. The representative then laboriously explained, with many diagrams, precisely how the steam engine worked. One by one, the villagers came around. There was only one stalwart who shouted at them, "Are all you people as crazy as the city people? For thousands of years, wagons never moved without horses, and now you believe there is some kind of magic that moves wagons without horses! We sent this man to the city, and the city people must have hypnotized him to believe in this fantasy, and you are foolish enough to go along with it!"

By this time the villagers had come around to understanding how the steam engine worked, so they all ganged up on this man, each one demonstrating convincingly how steam pressure can push a piston that turns the wheels. After a long discussion, the stalwart finally said, "Oh! Now I see. Of course, the steam pushes the piston and it turns the wheels. How simple!"

Everyone breathed a sigh of relief. The representative then addressed the group. "Does anyone have any further questions?"

The stalwart raised his hand. "I understand everything perfectly -- the steam pressure, the piston, the wheels. It's all very clear. I have only one question: on the diagram you made of that wagon, just where do you hitch up the horses?"

An open-minded person may not grasp something at first, but with a bit of explanation will understand it. If, after adequate explanation a person still cannot understand your point, he probably has his mind made up and will not yield regardless of how convincing you may be. Instead of exhausting yourself in futility, just assume that he won't get it.

But be careful! Don't allow another person's close-mindedness to get you in trouble. That's what happened to the next poor fellow:

In the horse-and-buggy days, a traveler alighted from the train and hired a taxi. He gave the driver his destination and said, "Be sure to avoid that one road. There's a deep ditch there."

The driver said, "Look, mister. I've been driving these roads for 35 years. Just sit back and relax."

A short while later, the passenger said, "You're traveling toward that road! Keep away from it. There's a big ditch there." The driver responded, "Didn't I tell you that I've been driving these roads for 35 years? Don't worry."

As they turned down the road, the passenger said, "Turn back! You're heading for the ditch." The driver said, "I've told you twice, I've been driving these roads for 35 years."

Sure enough, they fell into the ditch, horse and wagon on top of them. As the driver emerged from beneath the wagon, he said, "Funny thing! I've been driving these roads for 35 years, and whenever I come by here, this is what happens!"

Close-mindedness is just one kind of obstinacy. There is another variety of obstinacy in people who are forever discontented. Read on.

NEVER SATISFIED

A young man consulted me. He was completing his first of three years in radiology residency, but was dissatisfied with this area of medicine. He was thinking about either psychiatry or pathology, and wanted my opinion about which to choose.

I thought, "That's strange. Psychiatry or pathology? You couldn't possibly get two specialties that are more polar opposites. Psychiatry requires intense interpersonal relationships, whereas pathology has none at all."

The young man went on to say that prior to radiology he was in an internal medicine program, but he was not happy with that.

This aroused my suspicion. I asked, "Before medical school, were you in any other field?" He told me that he had started engineering, but had dropped it because he was not pleased with it.

"How did you manage to stay in medical school?" I asked.

"My family would have killed me if I had quit," he responded.

I then thought of a story that I had heard from my mother forty years earlier, but it had never come to mind before.

My mother used to tell me bedtime stories. She did not have a large repertoire, so she told the same stories over and over. But what of it? It wasn't the stories that counted. It was my mother's presence.

The story is about a stonecutter who earned his living hewing slabs of stone from a mountain. He often bewailed his sorry fate. "I have to work from dawn to dusk, breaking my back lifting this heavy pick-axe all day, and then I barely earn enough to put bread on the table for my family."

One day he heard a loud tumult. Climbing to the peak of the mountain, he could see from afar that there was a parade in the city. The king was in a royal procession, and people had lined the streets shouting "Bravo! Long live the king!" and throwing flowers at the royal coach.

The stonecutter raised his eyes to heaven "Dear Lord," he said, "You are a just God. That king and I are both human beings. Where is the justice that he should be so mighty and powerful, and I should be so downtrodden? If You are indeed just, You will give me the opportunity to be mighty as the king."

Suddenly, he felt himself transformed. God had answered his prayer. He was the mighty king, receiving accolades from thousands of loyal subjects. How thrilling it was to be so powerful!

But then he began to feel very uncomfortable. Clad in his ermine robe, he was wilting as the sun's rays fell upon him. "What!" he said. "The sun can humble a king? Then the sun is most powerful. I wish to be the sun."

He was transformed into the sun, and enjoyed its unequaled power. But then he found himself frustrated. A dark cloud had passed beneath him and was not allowing his rays to go through.

"What!" he said. "A cloud can frustrate the sun? Then it must be more mighty than the sun. I wish to be a cloud."

As a cloud, he took great pleasure in frustrating the sun, but then a sharp gust of wind blew him away. "The wind must be mightier than a cloud. I wish to be the wind."

As a wind, he became ferocious, causing tidal waves and leveling forests. But suddenly he was stymied. He had encountered a tall mountain which resisted his strongest gusts. "If a mountain is mightier than the wind, I wish to be a tall mountain."

As a tall mountain he dwarfed all else on earth, and felt most powerful. But then he felt a sharp pain. A stonecutter wielding a pick-axe was tearing away parts of him. He said, "If a stonecutter can dismantle a mountain, then he must be even mightier than the mountain, I wish to be that stonecutter."

And so he became the mightiest of all: a stonecutter.

I had not thought of that story until this young man told me how he was dissatisfied with everything he had been. I told him the story and said, "If you will be happy with yourself as a person, then you can be happy being an engineer or whatever kind of doctor you choose to be. If you are not happy with yourself, you can exhaust all the medical specialties and all the professions in the world and you will remain dissatisfied."

When I was five years old, I could not appreciate the wisdom in this bedtime story. It became apparent to me only forty years later.

A person with internal happiness can adjust to whatever position he attains. A person who seeks happiness in external sources may never be satisfied. He may be obstinate in making constant changes in the expectation of something that will relieve his discontent. Each change brings but a fleeting relief, and he may exhaust himself in a futile search for happiness.

IT'S HOW YOU SEE IT

Understandably, people do not consult a psychiatrist because of the good things that happen to them. They generally bring in a litany of hardships and setbacks they have suffered. Many times the psychiatrist may feel that the patient indeed has every right to be depressed.

My father taught me that mood may often depend on one's perspective rather than on the facts. He told me that in the villages of the old country, many people were illiterate. If they needed to write a letter, they would go to the town scribe.

One woman, whose son had emigrated to America, had not heard from him for several months. She asked the scribe to write a letter for her, and she dictated the following:
Dear Son:

I'm sorry that I have not heard from you for several months. Please write me and let me know how things are going for you.

With me, things are quite well. We have had a difficult winter, and the cold wind would come in through the crevices in the wall. But thank God, I was able to seal the crevices with old garments. The price of food has gone up very high, but thank God, day-old bread is much cheaper. I can afford this and I don't go hungry. I still have my house-cleaning job, and thank God that at my age I can still do this kind of work.

I am anxiously waiting to hear from you.
Love, Mother

The woman then asked the scribe to read what he had written. The scribe, who was outraged at the son's neglect of his elderly mother, wrote the following:
Dear Son:

What in the world is wrong with you that you have not written to me?

Conditions here are intolerable. The icy wind blows through the crevices in the walls, and I have to try to stuff them with rags. I can't afford proper food, and I have to survive on stale bread. At my old age I still have to get down on my hands and knees to scrub floors in order to survive. This is the kind of life I am leading here while you seem to be enjoying yourself in America.

When the scribe finished reading the letter, the woman grabbed hold of her head with both hands and said, "Oh, my God! I never knew how bad off I was until now!"

My father said, "The facts did not change. The same facts which had evoked a feeling of being fortunate now evoked a feeling of misery. It is not the facts in life that make the difference, but how you look at them."

TO WIN AN ARGUMENT

Having a "type A" personality, I must exert restraint to avoid interrupting people who are speaking to me. This is especially difficult in an argument, where the urge to promptly rebut my opponent is overwhelming. A story by Rabbi Nachman of Bratslav has helped me immensely.

A merchant was on his way home from the market when a highwayman accosted him and demanded his money at gunpoint. The merchant said, "Don't shoot!" and handed over his bag of money.

The merchant said to the robber, "I've given you all my money. Now I need a favor from you. My wife accuses me of gambling away my money, and she will never believe me that I was robbed. Please shoot a bullet through my hat, and I'll have proof that I was robbed."

The robber shot through the man's hat. The merchant then said, "Look, you have all my money. Help me convince my wife that I was robbed and did not gamble away my money. Please shoot a few bullets through my coat. The robber complied with his request.

"Can't you make just a few more bullet holes for me?" the merchant said.

The robber shot once and said, "That's all the bullets I have," whereupon the merchant jumped and beat him, retrieving his money.

I found that if I let my opponent "shoot all his bullets," I am in a much better position to triumph than if I were to interrupt and rebut his arguments when he still has some ammunition.

In a battle, allowing the enemy to exhaust his ammunition allows you to counterattack fearlessly. The same technique can be successful in an argument. If you are really interested in winning, you will use this technique.

THE WAY OF BUREAUCRACY

When I served on the Governor's Committee for Alcohol and Drugs, I attended meetings in the State Capitol. One time, a proposal for a project was presented which took the simplest idea and developed it into a confusing complexity. Every committee member was asked his opinion on the proposal. When my turn came, I said, "Let me tell you a story about the wise men of Chelm" (take a look earlier at "Seeking an Identity").

One winter morning, the people of Chelm awoke to find that during the night there had been a snowfall that had spread a beautiful white carpet over the town. They were delighted by its pristine beauty. It then occurred to them that every morning, the beadle went from house to house summoning people to morning prayers, and with his big, klutzy feet he would trample the snow and ruin its beauty. This had to be avoided.

The townsfolk called an emergency meeting of the wise men, who concluded that in order to prevent the beadle from trampling the snow, four men should carry the beadle from house to house.

"That ," I said, "is what this proposal sounds like."

Perhaps bureaucracy is not such a modern phenomenon after all.

THE PURSUIT OF HAPPINESS

The Founding Fathers said that among the inalienable rights of man are life, liberty and the pursuit of happiness. I have seen thousands of people pursue happiness, but they all seem to think it is somewhere else, when, in fact, it is actually within themselves. Ironically, their pursuit may take them away from the happiness they are seeking rather than toward it.

A rabbi once stopped a man who was hurrying in the marketplace. The man said, "I'm sorry, rabbi, I can't stop to talk with you now," he said. "I am in pursuit of my livelihood."

The rabbi said, "How do you know that your livelihood lies in the direction toward which you are going? Perhaps it is in the opposite direction, and you are running from it."

There is a story of a peasant who lived in a small village, who had a repetitive dream that under the foundation of a bridge in Prague, there lies buried a huge treasure. In spite of his wife's protests, he left for Prague. After several weeks of walking and hitch-hiking, he arrived in Prague and located the bridge. However, there were sentries on guard and he could not start digging. He sauntered around, looking for a time when the sentries might not be watching. Eventually, one of the sentries asked him, "Why are you constantly loitering here?"

The man decided to tell him the truth about his repetitive dream of the treasure buried under the bridge. The sentry howled with laughter. "And for that you came all the way here? Why, I have had a repetitive dream that under the floor of a peasant's hut in your village there is buried a huge treasure. Do you think I am foolish enough to go there to look for it?"

The man returned home, lifted the floorboards of his hut and found the treasure.

This folk tale, common to many cultures, indicates an awareness that we may often futilely look elsewhere for something we already have, but are unaware of. We seem to assume that if we are dissatisfied, we must look to some other place for satisfaction. Few people look within themselves, and may spend a lifetime in the "pursuit of happiness" when, in fact, they may actually be running from it.

Perhaps we should distinguish between pleasure and happiness. Many people confuse the two, and when they lack pleasure, they assume that they cannot be happy. The extreme of this error can be seen in the drug addict, whose only happiness seems to be in the euphoria of drugs that destroy his brain. This pathological pleasure eventually results in misery, if not death.

When I was a child, my mother told me a story which I came to appreciate only many years later. A poor man made a wish that he would have a purse which would never be empty. He found a magic purse which contained a dollar. When he removed the dollar, another came in its place. He was overjoyed that he would never be poor again, and kept on extracting dollars. Several days later he was found dead, lying atop of a huge pile of dollars. This is the "happiness" of addiction.

Happiness can be the result of self-fulfillment. If a person has a true self-awareness and strives to fulfill himself, he can be happy even if he does not have the ephemeral pleasures in which many people indulge.

There are so many things we can appreciate. Every day there is a sunset. Some of the sunsets are breathtakingly beautiful, and often are visible from our own porches.

The sound of the birds singing, the smell of freshly cut grass, the trees in spring blossom, the might and power of a thunderstorm, the smile on an infant's face, relaxing to the sound of music; all these and many more things at our fingertips can be sources of happiness.

A blind man was standing on a street corner with a cup which had only a few coins in it. A passerby wrote a little note and affixed it to the cup. It read, "Today is a beautiful spring day, and I am blind." Soon passers-by filled his cup.

I came across a poem from an unknown author that I would like to share with you.

> The park bench was deserted as I sat down to read
> Beneath the long, straggly branches of an old willow tree.
> Disillusioned by life with good reason to frown,
> For the world was intent on dragging me down.
>
> And if that weren't enough to ruin my day,
> A young boy out of breath approached me, all tired from play.
> He stood right before me with his head tilted down
> And said with great excitement, "Look at what I found."
>
> In his hand was a flower, and what a pitiful sight,
> With its petals all worn — not enough rain, or too little light.
> Wanting him to take his dead flower and go off to play,
> I faked a small smile and then shifted away.
>
> But instead of retreating he sat next to my side,
> And placed the flower to his nose and declared with overacted surprise,
> "It sure smells pretty and it's beautiful, too.
> That's why I picked it; here, it's for you."
>
> The weed before me was dying or dead,.
> Not vibrant of colors, orange, yellow or red.
> But I knew I must take it, or he might never leave.
> So I reached for the flower, and replied, "Just what I need."

But instead of him placing the flower in my hand,
He held it midair without reason or plan.
It was then that I noticed for the very first time
That weed-toting boy could not see: he was blind.

I heard my voice quiver, tears shone like the sun
As I thanked him for picking the very best one.
You're welcome," he smiled, and then ran off to play,
Unaware of the impact he'd had on my day.

I sat there and wondered how he managed to see
A self-pitying woman beneath an old willow tree.
How did he know of my self-indulged plight?
Perhaps from his heart, he'd been blessed with true sight.

Through the eyes of a blind child, at last I could see
And for all of those times I myself had been blind,
The problem was not with the world; the problem was me.
I vowed to see the beauty in life, and appreciate every second that's mine.

And then I held that wilted flower up to my nose
And breathed in the fragrance of a beautiful rose
And smiled as I watched that young boy, another weed in his hand
About to change the life of an unsuspecting old man.

  We need only to be reminded of our blessings to find happiness within our reach in everyday experiences. . . if we are not blind to them!